4

CW01521931

New Antibody Technology and the Emergence of Useful Cancer Therapy

edited by
Richard Begent and Anne Hamblin

Proceedings of the Tufton Trust Conference held at the Royal Society of Medicine on the 10th and 11th of October 1994

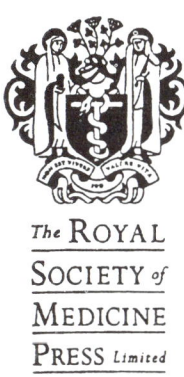

The ROYAL
SOCIETY *of*
MEDICINE
PRESS *Limited*

British Library Cataloguing-in-Publication Data

A catalogue record for this book is available from the British Library.

ISBN 1-85315-250-1

Cover picture:
Gamma camera image showing concentration of radiolabelled
antibody to CEA in a liver metastasis of colon carcinoma
in a patient receiving radioimmunotherapy.

Phototypeset by Dobbie Typesetting Limited, Tavistock, Devon
Printed in Great Britain by Page Bros. of Norwich

Editors and Co-Chairman

Professor Richard Begent
Cancer Research Campaign Targeting and Imaging Group,
The Royal Free Hospital School of Medicine, London, UK

Dr Anne Hamblin
Royal Veterinary College, London, UK

Speakers

Dr P. L. Amlot
Departments of Clinical Immunology and Clinical Oncology,
The Royal Free Hospital School of Medicine, London, UK

Professor K. Bagshawe
Emeritus Professor of Medical Oncology, Charing Cross and
Westminster Medical School, London, UK

Dr K. Chester
Cancer Research Campaign Targeting and Imaging Group,
The Royal Free Hospital School of Medicine, London, UK

Dr Anthony Cullen (Co-Chairman)
Vice President of the Royal Society of Medicine

Dr L. Durrant
Cancer Research Campaign Department of Clinical
Oncology, University of Nottingham, City Hospital,
Nottingham, UK

Dr A. A. Epenetos
Imperial Cancer Research Fund Department of Clinical
Oncology, Hammersmith Hospital, London, UK

Dr A. Griffiths
Medical Research Council Centre, Cambridge, UK

Dr R. Hawkins
Centre for Protein Engineering and Department of Clinical
Oncology, Addenbrooke's Hospital, Cambridge, UK

Dr P. Hamann
Lederle Research Division, American Home Products, Pearl
River, New York, USA

Dr J. Kemshead
Imperial Cancer Research Fund, Paediatric and
Neuro-Oncology Group, Frenchay Hospital, Bristol, UK

Dr J. Ledermann
Department of Oncology, University College London
Medical School, London, UK

Dr K. Mosbach
Pure and Applied Biochemistry, Chemical Center,
University of Lund, Sweden

Dr J. Taylor-Papadimitriou
Imperial Cancer Research Fund, Epithelial Cell Biology
Laboratory, Lincoln's Inn Fields, London, UK

Dr O. W. Press
Department of Medicine and Biological Structure,
University of Washington and the Fred Hutchinson Cancer
Research Center, Seattle, Washington, USA

Professor A. Rees
School of Biology and Biochemistry, University of Bath, UK

Dr R. Reisfeld (Co-Chairman)
The Scripps Research Institute, N Torrey Pines Road, La
Jolla, California, USA

Dr P. Riva
Nuclear Medicine Department, Ospedale Maurizio Bufalini-
Cesena, Italy

Mr N. Sacks
St George's Hospital, Blackshaw Road, London, UK

Dr S. Sharma
Cancer Research Campaign Targeting and Imaging Group,
Department of Clinical Oncology, The Royal Free Hospital
School of Medicine, London, UK

Dr C. Springer
Cancer Research Campaign Centre for Cancer
Therapeutics, Institute of Cancer Research, Sutton,
Surrey, UK

Mr N. A. Theodorou
Charing Cross Hospital, Fulham Palace Road, London, UK

Dr R. Walker
University of Leicester, Breast Cancer Research Unit,
Clinical Sciences, Glenfield Hospital, Groby Road,
Leicester, UK

Mr H. White (Co-Chairman)
Harley Street, London, UK

Acknowledgment

This Conference has taken place through the generosity of Sir Christopher Wates in memory of his late wife, Jeanne. Her courage and vision allowed her to discuss plans for the original Conference before she died in May 1989. The initial plan to bring together some of the keenest and most experienced minds working at the frontiers of cancer research have been realised both in the initial Conference and the present Conference, 'New Antibody Technology and the Emergence of Useful Cancer Therapy'. In acknowledging the generosity of Sir Christopher Wates through the Tufton Charitable Trust we recall Lady Wates' courage, vision and love of humanity.

Contents

REPORT OF THE MEETING

INTRODUCTION

Current cancer therapy is almost wholly reliant on non-specific cytotoxic and radiation delivery. Whilst some tumours can be cured regularly by this approach, most cannot. Escalations in dose can on occasions overcome resistance, but at the expense of systemic toxicity. New approaches with myelotoxic dose escalations requiring 'rescue' have found their place in haematological malignancies but are not yet (and may never be) in regular use for the common epithelial malignancies. It is clear that new treatment strategies are required. Ideally these new strategies would give tumouricidal doses locally without major systemic toxicity.

Treatment based upon the use of monoclonal antibodies has the appeal of selectivity, and in the two decades since the development of hybridoma technology enormous interest and research has centred on developing useful cancer treatments. In reality, however, it has only been in the past two or three years that some useful landmark studies have shown that we are coming closer to realising this potential.

Monoclonal antibodies can be generated against tumour-specific or tumour-abundant antigens and achieve antitumour effects either by innate mechanisms (complement or antibody dependent cytotoxicity, activation of immune mechanisms and growth factor inhibition) or by conjugation to an effector mechanism (toxin, radionuclide, activating enzyme or chemotherapeutic agent). However, a multitude of obstacles to effective therapy have been found when attempting to translate successes in cell culture and animal models to humans. Strategies to overcome these hurdles have been developed and have resulted in a radical rethink in many aspects of antibody-based therapy.

The main remit of the Tufton Charitable Trust conference held at the Royal Society of Medicine 10–11 October 1994 was to present and discuss recent technological achievements which have brought antibody-based therapy to the forefront of cancer treatment and to consider future directions.

This review will focus on the advances in technology and therapy presented at this conference.

NEW TECHNOLOGIES

One of the limitations of antibody technology has been the lack of specificity to human antigens. Hybridoma technology has enabled production of antibodies with specificities for various antigens by fusion of B-cells from an immunised animal with a mouse myeloma cell line. However, murine monoclonal antibodies lead to an antiglobulin response and hypersensitivity, thereby limiting their repeated use. Human monoclonal antibodies have a larger potential for repeated therapy but are difficult to make by immortalising B-lymphocytes and production of antibodies against human antigens is restricted by immune tolerance.

The human immune system has a large repertoire of (10^{12}) B cells, each containing unique antibody variable region (V) genes, that encode the specificity of the antibody on its cell surface. Exposure to and subsequent binding of an antigen, triggers differentiation into plasma cells that secrete antibody and memory cells that persist in the reticuloendothelial system. The V genes of these antibodies displayed on memory cells are subject to somatic mutation, leading to improved binding affinity after further exposure to antigen. The generation of large libraries of antibody V genes and the expression of these in filamentous bacteriophage has made it possible to mimic this system so that the diversity of the antibody response can be explored to produce antibodies for a desired clinical use.

In 1990, McCafferty et al. [1] demonstrated that a functional antibody fragment could be expressed on the surface of bacteriophage into which antibody V genes have been inserted. In this way the B-cell of the immune system is mimicked in a form in which the V genes and antibody expression can be readily manipulated. Combinatorial libraries can be constructed using filamentous bacteriophage from immunised animals by rearrangement of heavy and light chain V genes.

Immunisation may also be bypassed; peripheral blood lymphocytes from non-immunised donors can be used to provide a diverse source of rearranged V genes. The polymerase chain reaction is used to amplify the V_H and V_L families which can then be combined at random to

1

generate single chain Fv fragments which are cloned and displayed on the surface of phage [2].

Opening the meeting, Dr Griffiths described such a method for production of synthetic antibody repertoires. Antibody fragments are displayed on the surface of filamentous bacteriophage, each displaying an individual antibody. The phage are then selected by binding to antigen, and soluble antibody fragments are secreted from infected bacteria. The V genes are subjected to random mutation, allowing selection of mutants with higher affinities. Fragments with defined specificity against both foreign and self-antigens can be selected.

The larger the library, the greater the chance of finding antibodies that bind to any given epitope and the higher the affinity. The limiting factor is the efficiency of introduction of plasmid or phage DNA into bacteria. This can be improved by combinatorial infection generating more chain combinations.

Synthetic libraries of V_H and V_L can be used to generate new antibodies of improved specificity by an alternative method called chain shuffling. In this method the desired antigen binding site can be expanded by shuffling the individual V_H and V_L genes against libraries of light and heavy genes respectively. The best combination is then selected by binding with the original antigen, thus optimising pairing for specific antigen recognition.

The selection of such antibodies is critical. Filamentous phage can be used in selection. Dr Chester described a method by which phage technology was used to construct a library from B-cells of a mouse immunised with CEA (carcinoembryonic antigen). Rounds of selection were then performed in which phage reacting with antigen were bound to biotinylated CEA and then captured with streptavidin on a solid support. This identified clones with high affinity. A single clone—MFE23—was isolated, sequenced and antibody expressed in *Escherichia coli*. This antibody was found to be of very high affinity. It has now been purified and radiolabelled and used in clinical imaging trials. Should these confirm its superiority then it would be an ideal agent for use in genetically engineered antibody constructs for antibody-targeted therapy of cancer.

The ability to produce antibodies of enhanced affinity should improve as new technologies are used to increase the size and diversity of libraries. The availability of cloned human V_H, $V\kappa$ and $V\lambda$ gene segments, and knowledge about the structures they encode will allow the design of maximum structural diversity in primary repertoires. It should also allow the creation of premutated genes for use in making secondary repertoires in which mutations are focused at the antigen contacts or at sites likely to modulate the contacts.

Another technique for improving antibody diversity is molecular modelling. Detailed knowledge of existing antibody structures has shown that diversity of antibody binding sites is created during assembly of the V gene segments. In V_H the first two hypervariable loops are fairly well conserved but the third is variable in both sequence and length. V_L is similar with most of its diversity being derived from the third hypervariable loop although to a lesser extent than V_H.

Repeated therapy with mouse monoclonal antibodies causes an anti-antibody immune response which prevents repeated treatments. This can be largely overcome by replacing the murine constant regions with their human counterparts, a process known as humanisation. In addition, murine complementarity determining regions (cdrs)—the section of the antibody variable region which contains the antigen binding site—can be engrafted onto a human variable framework, retaining specificity and binding avidity of antigen, however, additional amino acid changes in the framework region are usually required to enable satisfactory binding.

Professor Rees described an alternative method by which only the surface residues of the murine framework, which are expected to cause immunogenicity, are replaced with alternative residues which are predicted to give a non-immunogenic structure. This is known as resurfacing.

Professor Rees also described how detailed analysis of the structure of both murine and human antibodies, has enabled families of V_L and V_H sequences to be identified. From these data the structure of other antibodies can be predicted. Changing specificity of an antibody is possible by *de novo* design. Side chains can be removed from the backbone and the antigen docked into the generic site, the side chains can then be reconstructed using knowledge about the three-dimensional structure. The best predications can then be incorporated into a phage library and the binding affinities compared. Thus entirely new antibodies with improved specificities can be generated.

Dr Mosbach described an alternative method for production of novel antigen binding molecules known as molecular imprinting. This depends on the creation of synthetic polymers with selective recognition sites. Functional monomers are polymerised in the presence of the molecule to be recognised which acts as a template resulting in a polymer with recognition sites which are imprints of the template. These polymers show a high degree of selectivity. The potential applications of the products of this technique are widespread and include the separation and purification of various biomolecules, stereo-isotopes and epitopes. The polymers produced to date have shown reactivity profiles similar to monoclonal antibodies.

ADVANCES IN RADIOIMMUNOTHERAPY

Monoclonal antibodies linked to beta- and alpha-emitting radionuclides can deliver therapy selectively to tumours when given intravenously or into body cavities. Beta-emitting radionuclides have a range of up to 400 cell diameters and this means that non-antigen-bearing tumour cells in the vicinity can also be killed. This is known as the 'bystander effect' and can overcome the problem of heterogeneity of antigen expression. It is also in this area of radioimmunotherapy that the most impressive successes of antibody targeted therapy have come.

Lymphoma is an appealing target given its innate radio-responsiveness and almost tumour-specific antigenic targets. Dr Press presented the experience of the Seattle group in the therapy of relapsed B-cell lymphoma. Their group uses an anti CD20 antibody linked to ^{131}Iodine(^{131}I), and treated 19 patients selected on favourable biodistribution with doses ranging from 280–777 mCi. This 'high dose' radioimmunotherapy required autologous bone marrow support but produced responses in 18 of the patients (16 of which were complete). The ongoing phase II study shows similar response rates but with toxicity less than that observed in standard bone marrow transplant conditioning regimens. CD20 would appear to be an excellent antigenic target as it is neither internalised nor shed after antibody binding. It is possible that this mode of therapy may replace external beam therapy in bone marrow transplant conditioning regimens. Kamiski *et al.* [3] and Bierman *et al.* [4] have also published reports supporting the promise of radioimmunotherapy in B-cell lymphoma and Hodgkin's disease respectively.

Radiolabelled antibody therapy has also shown effect in treatment of solid cancers whether given systemically or regionally, but radioresistance, intact host immune responses and poor tumour penetration has resulted in slower progress in this area.

The experience of intralesional therapy of high grade malignant glioma was reported by Dr Riva. Antibodies linked to ^{131}I targeting tenascin were injected into the cavity of gliomas after apparently complete resection or on recurrence. High tumour radiation doses were achieved (average 350 Gy per cycle) without local or systemic side effects. Responses were seen in 18 of 47 evaluable patients with median life expectancy improved from 12 to 18 months. Both Dr Riva and Dr Epenetos who spoke about radioimmunotherapy of ovarian cancer, focused on the remarkable success of this treatment in the adjuvant setting or in patients with small amounts of known tumour. Dr Epenetos reported on the work with HMFG1, a murine monoclonal antibody targeting polymorphic epithelial mucin (PEM) in patients with epithelial ovarian cancer. Intraperitonial administration was used, attempting to take advantage of the initial compartmental spread of this cancer. In the adjuvant setting (stages Ia to IV) enhanced survival was seen compared with a well documented regional control group. The possibility of other effector mechanisms (e.g. idiotypic vaccine) apart from the radionucleotide has been raised. A phase III trial in the adjuvant setting is now underway. This study, and one recently published by Riethmuller *et al.* [5] in colorectal cancer indicate the potential of antibody therapy in the adjuvant setting.

The regional therapy of meningeal tumours (either primitive neuroectodermal tumours or isolated central nervous system leukaemias) was reported by Dr Kemshead. The absence of human antimouse antibody (HAMA) in cerebrospinal fluid when it was present in blood allowed retreatment with antibody intrathecally and dose escalation. Because HAMA caused rapid blood clearance whilst having little effect on antibody clearance from the CSF, a differential between tumour and non-tumour absorbed doses was achieved. This tumour selectivity might be exploited in other regional treatment systems. Complete disappearance of disease and prolonged remissions were seen in these patients.

Professor Begent described his experience in radioimmunotherapy of colorectal cancer using antibodies targeting carcinoembryonic antigen (CEA). Therapeutic ratios of from 3:1 to 12:1 (tumour to bone marrow) have been achieved with response rates of 10% (similar to standard single agent chemotherapy regimens). Phosphor imaging of tumour cores after radiolabelled antibody therapy indicate the extent of heterogeneity of antibody distribution within tumour. It is not yet clear whether the bystander effect with radionuclides is sufficient to overcome this. Combining this treatment with tumour vascular modifiers (such as flavone acetic acid or methyl-4-xanthenone acetic acid) may potentiate treatment [6]. Antibody modification to increase affinity and thus tumour to normal tissue ratios and penetration as already described may also modify effect.

IMMUNOTHERAPY WITH ANTIBODY-CYTOKINE FUSION PROTEIN

Dr Reisfeld described a technique whereby an antibody was linked to interleukin-2 (IL-2). This entailed genetically engineering a human/mouse chimaeric antiganglioside GD2 antibody with recombinant human IL-2 (rhIL-2) by combining their genomic material for joint expression as one fusion protein by bacteria. He demonstrated that this fusion protein combined both antibody targeting ability with cytotoxic-directed effects of the cytokine molecule. This fusion protein was then administered to SCID mice with hepatic metastases from a human neuroblastoma tumour. The results demonstrated that the fusion protein was as effective as IL-2 alone in tumour cell lysis but the doses of IL-2 required were much smaller. This could have the therapeutic advantage of reducing the toxicity attributable to IL-2 in a clinical setting.

HUMAN RESPONSE TO ANTIBODIES

Antibody therapy to date has largely used murine monoclonal antibodies, which stimulate the production of HAMA. Once formed, HAMA complex with the antitumour antibody preventing tumour localisation and causing rapid clearance; there is also immediate type I or type III hypersensitivity in patients. Immunosuppressive drugs have been investigated to prevent HAMA formation, Dr Ledermann described the use of cyclosporin A which he has shown to delay the production of HAMA, allowing up to four courses of radioimmunotherapy to be delivered per patient.

Cyclosporin A is not without its toxicity. Various alternative methods have been used to prevent HAMA formation including chimeric antibodies and cdr grafting, resurfacing of antibodies as described by Professor Rees would also be an attractive alternative.

IMMUNOTOXINS AND CYTOTOXIC IMMUNOCONJUGATES

One of the limitations of antibody-targeted therapy is the small amount of therapeutic agent delivered to the tumour. This can potentially be overcome by the use of potent drugs and toxins which if used alone give unacceptable toxicity, conjugated to antibodies for selective tumour targeting. Internalisation of the antigen-antibody complex is required

to allow delivery of the toxic agent to the cancer cell DNA or ribosome for effect. The calicheamicin family of cytotoxic agents is one such group. These bind to the minor groove of DNA resulting in DNA cleavage and show potent antitumour activity on initial screening. Dr Hamann presented the preclinical development of calicheamicins conjugated to monoclonal antibodies targeting PEM in ovarian and breast cancer and CD33 in acute myelogenous leukaemia. Rapid internalisation of the antigen-antibody-drug complex is necessary and the antibodies were chosen with this in mind. Design of the linker between the antibody and calicheamicin is critical to allow unchanged internalisation and hydrolytic cleavage within the cancer cell. The uses of these drugs has some possible advantages over the use of immunotoxins as they are not expected to be immunogenic in man. The first clinical trial in acute myelogenous leukaemia is planned to start in December 1994.

The clinical experience with the use of immunotoxins in which antibody is linked to plant toxins such as ricin A chain or saporin, has been clouded by the frequency of the potentially serious vascular leak syndrome (VLS) as explained by Dr Amlot. Responses, however, do occur, especially in lymphoid malignancies. Anti-antibody and anti-ricin formation, even in this inherently immuno-suppressed group, is a further problem. Their main advantage, despite this, is the low level of haematological toxicity and it is possible that the combination of immunotoxin with conventional cytotoxic agent may have a synergistic antitumour effect. The mode of action of ricin A chain based on ribosomal inhibitory proteins (and therefore protein synthesis inhibition) may overcome multidrug resistance. The future of immunotoxin therapy relies upon the production of smaller non-immunogenic molecules and the avoidance of VLS by dose optimisation. Bispecific antibodies relying on a two-stage approach in which antibody is targeted to tumour in the first phase and toxin is captured by antibody and internalised when given in a second phase may hold the key.

DIAGNOSTIC AND PROGNOSTIC FACTORS

Accurate diagnosis of the extent of tumours is critical in determining the adequacy of a surgical resection and the long-term outcome. Identification of certain tumour-associated antigens can be important for assessment of the likelihood of a tumour to respond to certain treatment as well as the overall prognosis. Current techniques for assessment of disease rely on imagining techniques which have limited resolution and analysis of histological specimens both by conventional analysis and immunohistochemistry.

Immunohistochemistry in which antigens can be detected within tissue sections or cells has become more widely available over the last 20 years. Frozen or fixed tissue can be used and smaller amounts of tissue can be analysed than with conventional biochemical techniques. Immunohistochemistry can give additional information such as the actual site of antigen localisation (e.g. oestrogen receptors) and the proportion of cells within a tumour that express the particular antigen. Problems arise with quantification of the amount of antigen present within a tissue, and whether this is present in an active or latent form. Dr Walker described the use of immunohistochemistry in breast cancer where it can be used to aid selection of the appropriate treatment, characterise the behaviour of the tumour and thereby predict prognosis. By identifying the presence of a particular tumour antigen immunohistochemistry may allow the patient to be treated by an antibody directed therapy and, in addition, if present in the serum, the antigen may be used to assess disease response and the likelihood of recurrence of the disease in longterm follow-up.

Currently immunohistochemistry can be used to identify which therapy is the best option with tumours showing positivity for oestrogen, and progesterone receptors responding better to endocrine manipulation; those which are positive for Ki 67—a marker of cellular proliferation— are more likely to respond to chemotherapy. Further information is derived from another tumour antigen c-erbB$_2$ which is overexpressed in 20–30% of invasive carcinomas and amplification of the corresponding DNA is correlated with overexpression of the protein and a poor prognosis.

The advantage of immunohistochemistry is that a wide range of antigens and antibodies are available for use on small tissue samples which may be fixed or fresh. It can be used for identifying specific antigens which can give information about both likelihood of response to certain types of therapy and prognosis. However, in order to improve the efficiency of this technique, the methods for identification of antigens must be standardised and quality control developed.

Antibodies to tumour antigens can also be used preoperatively for identifying tumour distribution. This can be done by using a radiolabelled antibody to a known tumour specific antigen. This assessment can be important with regard to the surgery performed. One example is in early invasive breast cancer where the problem lies with axillary node dissection. Axillary node dissection is performed for several reasons: to optimise tumour control without the need for radiotherapy and it's toxicity. The identification of tumour in axillary nodes establishes an independent risk factor for the development of metastatic disease and selecting those patients who benefit from adjuvant chemotherapy. The Early Breast Cancer Trialists' Collaborative Group in 1992 produced an overview of chemotherapy which demonstrated that longterm survival with six months of adjuvant therapy improves 10 year survival in node positive disease by 7% compared with 3% of node negative disease [7]. Mr Sacks described one such tumour antigen—c-erbB$_2$. This is an oncoprotein which is over-expressed in 20–30% of invasive breast cancer and is associated with a poor prognosis, increased risk of relapse, reduced disease-free survival and reduced overall survival.

Those patients whose tumours overexpress c-erbB$_2$ show a poor response to both endocrine manipulation and chemotherapy. C-erbB$_2$ has a low level of expression elsewhere in the body thereby making it a suitable target for antibody-directed therapy. His group have used such an antibody to c-erbB$_2$ in immunohistochemistry to demonstrate the presence of tumour in lymph nodes with an 80% accuracy compared with 66% seen with previous antibodies and 70% compared with clinical examination.

Mr Sacks has also demonstrated tumour regression using ^{131}I labelled antibody in nude mice bearing breast carcinoma xenografts overexpressing c-erbB$_2$. The antibody showed saturable binding and also diminished affinity with conjugation to radioisotope; it is, therefore, necessary to identify the minimum amount of radioactivity required. The use of clearing antibodies to remove background radioactivity and antibody fragments rather than the intact molecule to improve tumour penetration, may increase the efficiency of this system.

A further role for an antibody-directed approach is peroperatively. In colorectal carcinoma, surgery is the mainstay of treatment and the extent of primary resection is vital in establishing prognosis. Peroperative localisation of tumour may help to improve the accuracy of resection. Mr Theodorou described a trial where patients were given ^{125}I labelled anti-CEA (A5B7) 4–16 days prior to surgery. A hand-held gamma-detecting probe was then used at operation to identify tumour at resection margins and guide to the extent of resection required. A5B7 and its F(ab')2 fragment have both been used and shown to localise well to tumour. The sensitivity was 95% and accuracy rate was 57% with additional clinical information gained in primary resections in 27% and changing the management in 9%. In second look operations the management was altered in 39%. It was difficult to identify lymph node involvement due to the high background radiation and distortion by the primary tumour; this method can measure masses as small as 0.1 g but can miss very small secondaries; the numbers of false negatives is 12%. Ideally the antibody should be taken up rapidly by all deposits and have a high tumour to normal tissue ratio. *Ex vivo* examination of the lymph nodes has been shown to improve the degree of accuracy—G. L. Smith *et al.* (poster 13) studied 30 lymph nodes from 11 patients using a CC49 anti-TAG72 antibody. The accuracy was 80% which was equivalent to immunohistochemistry using conventional anti-CEA antibodies.

VACCINES

An alternative approach to the antibody-directed therapies described previously would be to recruit the host's immune system in some way to effectively destroy tumour cells.

Many tumours express tumour-associated antigens on their surface which can be recognised by T-cells. They are not however, immunogenic in the recognised manner because they fail to induce an immune response.

The failure of recognition is probably due to several mechanisms including the way in which the antigen is presented to the T-cell and the lack of co-stimulatory molecules.

In order to produce a tumour-specific response, the antigen selected must be present either exclusively on tumour cells or have different epitopes to the equivalent molecule on normal cells. One such molecule is the polymorphic epithelial mucin (PEM). It is the product of the MUC1 gene, whose sequence has been identified. The PEM molecule is ideally suited to active specific immunotherapy for several reasons: it is overexpressed and upregulated by many cancers, the aberrant glycosylation exposes epitopes which are not present on mucin from normal cells; within each molecule are a series of tandem repeats, each containing several epitope sites. Most importantly, it does not require interaction with HLA system in order to activate T-cells. Dr Taylor-Papadimitriou discussed the use of PEM and its ability to produce both humoral and cellular responses. She also described both synergenic and transgenic mouse models for testing clinical response, toxicity and quantitative measurement of the immune response.

An antigen which is probably completely tumour-specific is that found on the surface of clonally expanded B-cells in B-cell lymphomas. This tumour is a good model for immunotherapy as each B-cell expresses an idiotypic immunoglobulin on its cell surface.

Immunisation with the idiotypic antibody has resulted in some good responses, but these are very few and limited by mutations in the immunoglobulins. Dr Hawkins described the use of plasmid DNA vaccination for immunotherapy in B-cell lymphomas. In this method tumour variable region genes were amplified using the polymerase chain reaction and heavy and light V genes linked. These were then expressed by plasmid vectors to allow high levels of transfection. Intramuscular immunisation with plasmid DNA results in production of the corresponding scFv and presentation by antigen presenting cells in such a way that immune tolerance to the idiotype specific to the lymphoma is broken. This has produced effective therapy in a mouse mode and a clinical trial is soon to begin.

Dr Durrant described an anti-idiotype vaccine for use in colorectal cancer. In the immune system, control of the production of antibodies to any particular antigen is carried out by a second antibody directed against the idiotype of the original antibody. This second antibody can have an epitope identical to that of the tumour antigen. A tumour-associated antigen is not normally immunogenic to the host but this second antibody, the anti-idiotype, is able to stimulate an immune response. The antibody described is a human monoclonal anti-idiotypic antibody, which mimics a colorectal tumour antigen and induces anti-colorectal tumour immune response in animals. Dr Durant's data showed induction of T-cell blastogenesis and enhanced IL-2 production. In Phase I clinical studies it was associated with no toxicity. The mechanisms were thought to be both via specific and non-specific effector mechanisms.

These methods, all utilising the host's own immune response to destroy tumours, offer a promising new addition to the antibody therapies currently available and a randomised trial of this antibody vaccine compared with conventional treatment of metastatic colorectal cancer is in progress.

ADEPT (Antibody Directed Enzyme Prodrug Therapy)

ADEPT is a novel approach to cancer therapy designed to overcome some of the limitations of conventional antibody therapy. This system relies on antibodies directed against tumour-associated antigens to target enzymes to cancer sites. When this complex is cleared from non-tumour sites a prodrug activated by the enzyme is given; this results in production of a cytotoxic drug locally in the tumour. The enzyme can continue to turnover prodrug thus amplifying the effect as well as allowing a tumour bystander effect against antigen-negative cancer cells. Internalisation of antibody is not necessary in this system and by using non-mammalian enzyme systems the prospect of non-specific prodrug activation is minimised. This concept is applicable to any tumour system which can be targeted and has the conceptual advantage of multiple prodrug/drug combinations to overcome drug resistance.

Professor Bagshawe described the theory and results of the first clinical trial of ADEPT in colorectal cancer. The F(ab′)2 fragment of A5B7 anti-CEA antibody was used to deliver the bacterial carboxypeptidase G2 enzyme to tumour. After clearance this would activate the mono-mesyl benzoic acid mustard drug CMDA (an alkylating agent was chosen as drug resistance can be overcome by dose escalation with this cytotoxic class). The trial design looked at a number of parameters including prodrug administration technique (bolus versus continuous infusion) and the influence of varying blood levels of antibody-enzyme conjugate. A further phase I trial with the same reagents is proceeding to further optimise the design of the ADEPT system. Whilst the patients treated had extremely advanced disease, responses were seen in five out of eight patients indicating the potential of this treatment strategy.

The ADEPT system has many variables which interact with each other. The design is therefore amenable to alteration at any level to optimise the system as a whole. Whilst numerous enzyme-prodrug systems have been described, the fundamentals of antibody design, affinity and tumour penetration still remain.

Dr Springer described how prodrug design and production could help to optimise the ADEPT approach. She was able to synthesise a range of different aromatic nitrogen mustard prodrugs by substituting at various points on the basic benzene ring. All had poor cytotoxic activity until cleaved by carboxypeptidase G2 thus fulfilling the first requirement as a prodrug.

A favourable prodrug was sought and it was thought that its profile should include (1) favourable enzyme kinetics, (2) a short active drug half-life (to reduce leak-back of active drug from the tumour to vulnerable normal tissues) and (3) increased potency of the active drug. A di-iodo phenol mustard prodrug has been developed which best

meets the target criteria and this is to go into the next clinical ADEPT trial.

Dr Sharma discussed some of the other fundamental changes which could help improve the ADEPT system. After localisation of the enzyme conjugate it is advantageous to accelerate clearance of enzyme conjugate from non-tumour sites. This would increase the therapeutic ratio and reduce non-tumour toxicity. Enzyme inactivation and accelerated clearance systems using second antibodies or a streptavidin-biotin system were described. Co-administration of vasoactive agents such as tumour necrosis factor alpha may increase tumour localisation. Repeated treatments of ADEPT are now possible using immunosuppressive techniques and as better agents for this purpose are identified, the system might be easier to administer.

Whilst ADEPT in its current form remains complex, its potential application in colorectal and other cancers is enormous. Current advances in antibody technology and targeting, enzyme-prodrug systems, tumour to non-tumour enzyme ratios and immunosuppression should markedly improve response rates.

CONCLUSION

Antibody-based technology is fulfilling its potential as a new cancer therapy. Radioimmunotherapy has already been shown to produce sustained complete responses in B-cell lymphomas [8] and also gives responses in other malignancies. This conference has described some of the new and exciting prospects emerging in this field. Antibodies are versatile and can be used in a multitude of ways; as a diagnostic tool, combined with various therapeutic modalities, in an adjuvant setting and as vaccines.

There has been an enormous expansion in the methodology for the production of antibodies with improved specificity and binding affinities. This technology combined with production of anti-idiotypic antibodies and upregulation of the host's immune system can create a framework for the future direction of antibody therapy. Such advances in expertise make cancer cure a realistic goal.

K. Eagle and **M. P. Napier**
Department of Clinical Oncology,
The Royal Free Hospital,
Pond Street, London NW3 2QG, UK

REFERENCES

1 McCafferty J, Griffith AD, Winter G, Chiswell D. Phage antibodies: filamentous phage displaying antibody variable domains. *Nature* 1990; *348*: 552–4

2 Marks JD, Hoogenboom HR, Bonnert TP, *et al.* By-passing immunisation–human antibodies from V-gene libraries displayed on phage. *J Mol Biol* 1991; *222*: 581–97

3 Kaminsky MS, Zasadny KR, Francis IR, *et al.* Radio-immunotherapy of B-Cell Lymphoma with 131-I Anti B1 (Anti-CD20) Antibody. *N Engl J Med* 1993; *329*: 459–65

4 Bierman PJ, Vose JM, Leichner PK, *et al.* Yttrium 90–labelled antiferritin followed by high dose chemotherapy and autologous bone marrow transplantation for poor–prognosis Hodgkin's disease. *J Clin Oncol* 1993; *11*: 698–703

5 Riethmuller G, Schneider-Gadicke E, Schlimok G, *et al.* Randomised trial of monclonal antibody for adjuvant therapy of resected Duke's C colorectal cancer. *Lancet* 1994; *343*: 1177–83

6 Pedley RB, Begent RHJ, Boden JA, *et al.* Enhancement of radioimmunotherapy by drugs modifying tumour blood flow in a colonic xenograft model. *Int J Cancer* 1994; *57*: 830–5

7 Early Breast Cancer Trialist's Collaborative Group. Systemic treatment of early breast cancer by hormonal, cytotoxic or immune therapy. *Lancet* 1992; *339*: 1–15, 71–86

8 Press OW, Eary JF, Appelbaum FR, *et al.* Radiolabelled-Antibody Therapy of B-Cell Lymphoma with Autologous Bone Marrow Support. *N Engl J Med*; *329*: 1219–24

Isolation of high affinity human antibodies directly from large phage-display libraries

Andrew David Griffiths

MRC Centre for Protein Engineering, MRC Centre, Hills Road, Cambridge, UK

The mammalian immune system can generate antibodies with high affinities and exquisite specificities for antigens. However, it has evolved to provide a defence against invading pathogens and will frequently not produce antibodies with the optimal characteristics required for research, industrial or medical applications.

A particular problem is with antibodies intended for therapeutic use in humans. Monoclonal antibodies (mAbs) are traditionally made by immortalising B-lymphocytes from an immunised donor to create cell lines secreting antibodies with a single specificity. Although rodent mAbs are easy to produce using this 'hybridoma technology', when used therapeutically in humans they are frequently recognised as foreign, leading to complications which necessitate the termination of treatment.

Human mAbs are, therefore, the ideal choice for therapy. Unfortunately, antigen-driven expansion of B-lymphocyte clones is important for the generation of mAbs by immortalisation. Immunological tolerance mechanisms normally prevent expansion of B-cell clones with self-specificities. Thus, it is very difficult to generate human mAbs directed against human antigens (self-antigens). This is a serious limitation as many of the most promising targets for therapeutic antibodies are self-antigens.

In addition, immunisation of human subjects with foreign antigens is frequently not possible (or at least not ethical), as is the case, for example, with highly toxic substances or cancer cells. Even where an immunised donor is available there are many technical difficulties associated with making human mAbs.

To avoid these problems we have created an *in vitro* system for the generation of human mAbs without immunisation, based on the selection of antibody libraries displayed on filamentous phage.

Such libraries can be constructed using antibody variable region genes (V-genes) from unimmunised human donors or from synthetic antibody V-genes constructed *in vitro*. We have shown that such a 'single-pot repertoire' can provide antibodies with exquisite specificities for many different antigens [1]. However, the affinities of the antibodies are only moderate ($\sim \mu M$), but can be improved by further rounds of mutation and selection.

It would obviously be advantageous to be able to isolate high affinity antibodies directly from phage-display libraries. We speculated that one way to do this would be to create larger repertoires than those existing at present, which are limited in size to a maximum of about 10^8 by transformation efficiency.

To this end we have generated a system for the production of very large phage-antibody repertoires. We first created highly diverse repertoires of heavy and light chains entirely *in vitro* from a bank of human V-gene segments and cloned the heavy and light chain genes onto separate vectors. The heavy and light chain genes were then recombined onto the same replicon, within bacterial cells, using the loxP-Cre recombination system of bacteriophage P1, to generate a large (6.5×10^{10}) synthetic repertoire of Fab fragments displayed on filamentous phage. From this repertoire we isolated Fab fragments which bound to a range of different antigens and haptens, and with binding affinities comparable to those of antibodies from a secondary immune response in mice (up to 4 nM) [2]. Although the V_H-26 (DP-47) segment was the most commonly used segment in both artificial and natural repertoires, there were also major differences in the pattern of segment usage. Such comparisons may help dissect the contributions of biological mechanisms and structural features governing V-gene usage *in vivo*.

We believe that the ability to produce antibodies of high affinity directly from a single repertoire makes this technology, at the very least, highly competitive with existing monoclonal antibody technology and in many cases, especially for the production of human monoclonal antibodies (for therapy), it may even show some distinct advantages.

REFERENCES

1 Winter G, Griffiths AD, Hawkins RE, Hoogenboom HR. Making antibodies by phage display technology. *Annu Rev Immunol* 1994; *12*: 433–55

2 Griffiths AD, Williams SC, Hartley O, *et al*. Isolation of high affinity human antibodies directly from large synthetic repertoires. *EMBO J* 1994; *13*: 3245–60

Antibody structure and design

Anthony R. Rees, Graham Elliott and Sue Phillips
School of Biology and Biochemistry, University of Bath, Bath, UK

INTRODUCTION

At the time of writing the Brookhaven Protein Structural Database (established by Berstein *et al.* [1] and continuously updated) contains 45 or so structures of antibodies or their fragments (including complexes with antigen and light chain dimers) while about 2000 variable-region sequences have been determined (Kabat database [2]). The rate of sequence acquisition continues to outstrip the rate of structure determination and, although X-ray crystallography or nuclear magnetic resonance (NMR) spectroscopy are the preferred methods for producing structures at atomic resolution, the need for good three-dimensional models to guide antibody engineering has become essential. Such models will be increasingly useful for assessing the structural effects of point mutations within the antibody combining site, for designing minimal perturbation strategies for grafting complementarity-determining regions (humanization), and for rationally selecting residues on the basis of their likely accessibility to antigen that can be targeted for random mutation by gene library methods (e.g. 'phage libraries'). Where antibody specificity is modified 'by design', the three-dimensional structure or model will be not so much useful as essential.

ANTIBODY–ANTIGEN INTERACTIONS

The great majority of antibodies has been raised against protein or peptide antigens. The first attempt to improve the affinity of a monoclonal antibody *in vitro* used site-directed mutagenesis guided by crude models, and achieved and improvement in affinity of an order of magnitude [3]. Since these early experiments, modelling has improved to the point where the positions of complementarity-determining region (CDR) residues at or near the putative antigen-binding region can be more accurately specified. Methods of modelling antibody combing site are exemplified by the work of Chothia and Lesk [4] and Chothia *et al.* [5,6], for up to five of the six CDRs and, in a fully integrated software package, by Pedersen *et al.* [7], Searle *et al.* [8] and Rees *et al.* [9] for all six CDRs. Examples of where modelling can be used to improve the effectiveness of protein engineering experiments can be found in Sharon [10], Denzin *et al.* [11] and Kelly and O'Connell [12].

Given such methodological improvements, can the effects of mutations on affinity be predicted?

Inspection of antibody-protein crystal structures suggest that there is no obvious correlation between the number or type of interaction seen (such as van der Waals or hydrogen bonding or salt bridges) and affinity. In addition, the buried surface area is not a good indicator of affinity, although this might be the case if burial of hydrophobic residues and release of water molecules were the major contributor to the free energy of binding. In fact, recent work by Poljak and co-workers [13] suggests the reverse. During measurements of the enthalpic and entropic contributions to the association of hen's egg lysozyme (HEL) with D1.3 using microcalorimetry, it was found that the binding was substantially enthalpically driven, while the entropy actually decreased. While this may not always be so, it is clear that the differing affinities observed in different complexes may have their origins in rather different profiles of interaction. A good fit of the two surfaces is clearly important for high affinity, but after this has been achieved, the thermodynamics may be driven by many different combinations of hydrophobic and electrostatic interactions. There is probably more of a balance between these two

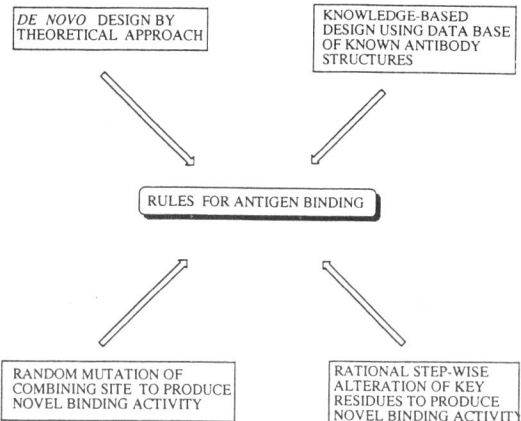

Figure 1. *De novo* design of antibody combining sites

randomisation (32 codons) within the context of a library of between 10^8 and 10^{10} recombinants. Although this can be improved by use of 'clustering' methods that reduce the 20 amino acids to groups of chemically similar members (e.g. Arkin *et al.* [14]), we have taken a more rational approach which explores the application of theoretical methods.

It is now possible to produce three-dimensional models of the antibody combining-site from CDR sequences alone. However, to generate an antibody specificity *de novo* requires that a particular set of CDR sequences must be predicted to give rise to particular antibody combining site shape. This process is by no means simple and is at the heart of the design concept. Our analysis of more than 70 antibodies for which the antigens are known has suggested that there is no strong relationship between particular

types of interaction than is evident in other protein-protein complexes since, for much of its life, the antibody must retain stability in the *absence* of any bound antigen.

Where does all this leave the antibody designer? Clearly, any redesign strategy must target both polar and non-polar residues in a way that, ideally, will lead to both enthalpic and entropic improvements in the interaction interface.

ANTIBODY DESIGN—A BLUEPRINT

The design or re-design of antibody specificity can be approached from either a purely theoretical direction, from the analysis of rationally or randomly mutated combining sites, or from a combination of both (Figure 1). Where random mutagenesis is contemplated, the number of positions that can be targeted will be limited by factors such as codon redundancy and transformation efficiency. These effects can be seen in Figure 2 to restrict the number of mutable positions to about five or six for complete

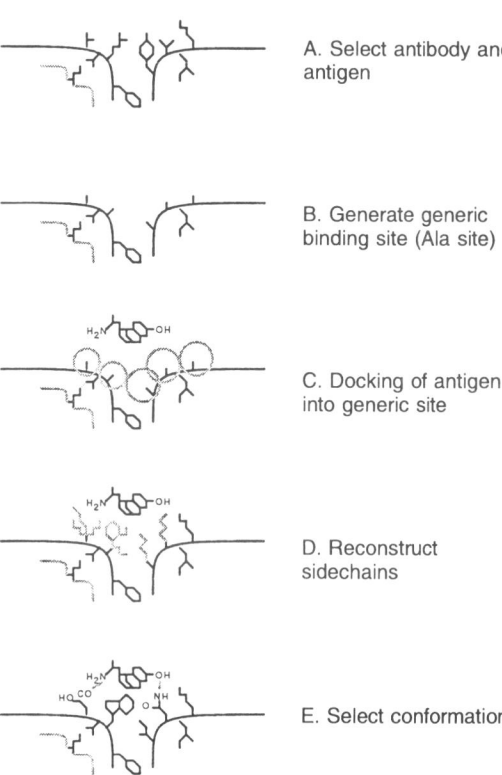

A. Select antibody and antigen

B. Generate generic binding site (Ala site)

C. Docking of antigen into generic site

D. Reconstruct sidechains

E. Select conformations

Figure 3. In the design process (outlined in detail in the text) an antibody of known structure is chosen by random. A generic (alanine) binding site is generated by replacing all non-structural residues by alanine with an extended VdW radius. A tentative docking is performed, and sidechains reconstructed. Using various objective scoring functions the sidechain conformations are evaluated, and a final conformation is selected.

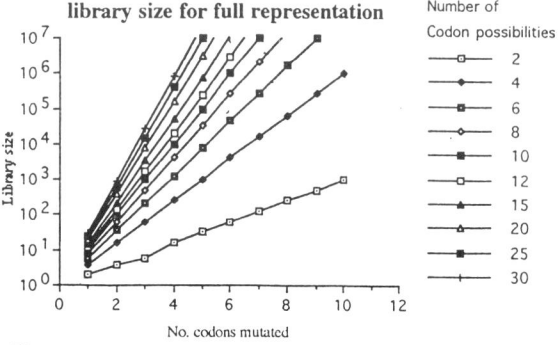

Figure 2.

combinations of CDR lengths and antigen size (Pedersen [15]). However, the coarse topography of a combining site (cavity, groove or planar class; see [16]) will be dictated by the backbone conformation, while the fine specificity for the epitope will largely be determined by the side chains. This leads to the hypothesis that any antibody in a given topographic class that is stripped of all those side chains that do not play a structural role should provide a combining site that is generic for a large number of different antigens.

These assumptions have led us to a design strategy that is now being tested. The concept is illustrated in Figure 3 and follows the sequence set out in the legend. This design process can be tested by synthesis and expression of candidate designs or by phage-library methods. Sequences identified as new antigen binders can then be analysed and fed back into the design process. When design algorithms like these are fully developed, they will take their places alongside the more traditional immunization and gene library methods *in vivo* and will probably in time become the method of choice where antigen structure is known.

Acknowledgments

We would like to thank BBSRC, British Biotechnology and the Wellcome Foundation for a LINK grant and Oxford Molecular, for the use of computer equipment.

REFERENCES

1 Bernstein FC, *et al.* Computer based archival file for macromolecular structure. *J Mol Biol* 1977; **112**: 535–42

2 Kabat E, Wu TT, Reid-Miller M, Perry HM, Gottesman KS, Foeller C. *Sequences of Proteins of Immunological Interest* (5th edn) US Department of Health and Human Services, USA, 1992

3 Roberts S, Cheetham HC, Rees AR. Generation of an antibody with enhanced affinity and specificity for its antigen by protein engineering. *Nature* 1987; *328*: 731–4

4 Chothia C, Lesk AM. Canonical structures for the hypervariable regions of immunoglobulins. *J Mol Biol* 1987; **196**: 907–17

5 Chothia C, *et al.* The conformations of immunoglobulin hypervariable regions. *Nature* 1989; **342**: 877–83

6 Chothia C, *et al.* Structural repertoires of the human VH segments. *Mol Biol* 1992; **227**: 799–817

7 Pedersen JT, Searle SMJ, Henry AH, Rees AR. Antibody modelling: beyond homology. *Immunomethods* 1992 **1**: 126–36

8 Searle SMJ, Pedersen JT, Henry AH, Webster DM, Rees AR, Borrebaeck CAK, eds, *Antibody Structure and Function* Oxford University Press (in press)

9 Rees AR, Pedersen JT, Searle S. *AbM^TM, an integrated antibody modelling software suite.* Oxford Molecular plc, 1992

10 Sharon J. Structural correlates of high antibody affinity: three engineered amino acid substitutions can increase the affinity of an anti-p-azophenylarsonate antibody 200-fold. *Proc Natl Acad Sci USA* 1990; **87**: 4814–17

11 Denzin L K, Whitlow M, Voss EW, Jr. Single chain site-specific mutations of fluorescein amino acid contact residues in high affinity antibody 4-4-20. *J Mol Biol* 1991

12 Kelly RF, O'Connell. Thermodynamic analysis of an antibody functional epitope. *Biochemistry* 1993; **32**: 6828–35

13 Tello D, Goodbaum FA, Mariuzza RA, Ysern X, Schwarz FP, Poljak RJ. Three-dimensional structure and thermodynamics of antigen binding by anti-lysozyme antibodies. *Biochem Soc Transac* 1994; **21**: 943–6

14 Arkin AP, Youvan DC. Optimizing nucleotide mixtures to encode specific subsets of amino acids for semi random mutagenesis. *Bio/Technology* 1992; **10**: 297

15 Pedersen JT. Antibody combining sites. PhD Thesis, University of Bath, UK 1993

16 Webster DM, Henry AH, Rees AR. Antibody-antigen interactions. *Curr Opin Struct Biol 1994;* **4**: 123–9

Filamentous phage antibodies: the power of selection for clinical use

Kerry A. Chester, Richard H.J. Begent,
Lynda Robson, Patricia Keep, R. Barbara Pedley,
Joan A. Boden, Geoff Boxer, Alan Green,
Paul Michael, Greg Winter, Olivier Cochet
and Robert E. Hawkins
Royal Free Hospital School of Medicine, London, UK

The combinatorial library approach to antibody production allows generation of vast numbers of potentially clinically useful antibodies and a wide range of techniques are now available to create these libraries from murine, human or synthetic antibody genes. The larger the library and the greater the diversity the greater the chance of optimal antibodies being present, but unless a powerful selection method is available for the retrieval of a desired antibody this would be a task similar to that of isolating a needle from a haystack. The use of filamentous bacteriophage makes it possible to screen and select from libraries of hundreds of millions of antibody specificities. The libraries are constructed so that each phage expresses an antibody on its surface and contains the corresponding antibody gene [1]. Genes which encode antibodies with desired characteristics are then readily selected by reactivity of the phage with antigen (reviewed by Hawkins *et al.*, 1992 [2]). Here we describe how the system has been used to produce an antibody to carcinoembryonic antigen (CEA). This phage-derived antibody has higher affinity and better tumour specificity than anti-CEAs currently in use.

Radiolabelled antibody to CEA has been successful in imaging colorectal tumours and may be useful for therapy if the targeting efficiency could be improved [3]. Antibodies of higher affinity may achieve this [4] and improved tumour specificity would also be of value. To obtain a high affinity anti-CEA a combinatorial phage antibody library biased for antibodies reactive with CEA was first constructed. Mice were immunised with CEA (as for the production of conventional monoclonal antibodies) to achieve this because mRNA from the spleen of immunised animals is greatly enriched for the desired antibody genes and provides an appropriate starting point of CEA reactive variable regions. mRNA was extracted from splenic lymphocytes obtained from the immunised mice and the variable genes amplified with specific primers using the polymerase chain reaction (PCR). PCR amplified V_H and V_L were then randomly combined and assembled as single chain Fvs (scFvs) by PCR addition of overhanging oligonucleotides encoding the (glyglyglyglyser)x3 linker to tether the carboxy terminal end of V_H to the amino terminal end of V_L [5]. The products were cloned into the pHEN phagemid vector to produce a library of 10^7 scFvs [6].

To select an antibody with specificity and high affinity for CEA a method developed by Hawkins *et al.*, (1992)[7] was employed. The total phage library was allowed to bind biotinylated CEA and bound phage were subsequently captured with streptavidin coated beads. These selected phage were amplified in number by infection and overnight growth in *Escherichia coli*. Several rounds of selection were performed and the progress monitored by phage ELISA. A positive reaction with CEA was obtained after the first selection (O.D. 0.13 compared to 0.013 for the original library) and the strength of the signal increased with two successive rounds to O.D. 1.12. At this point individual clones were examined by DNA sequencing; of 24 clones sequenced at least nine different ones were identified showing that there were different anti-CEA antibodies present. To obtain a scFv which bound CEA at low concentrations (i.e. high affinity) two further rounds of selection were performed using a low concentration of biotinylated CEA (5 nM). The selected clones were then analysed individually and 34 of 50 clones were positive in ELISA. DNA sequencing revealed that the five with the strongest ELISA signal were from the same clone. This clone was named MFE-23.

MFE-23 was subcloned for expression as a soluble scFv linked to a C-terminal myc tag to aid identification during protein purification. Protein production (20–40 mg per litre) from cultures of bacteria was obtained after 24 h and the scFv was purified on CEA-Sepharose affinity chromatography and by size exclusion gel filtration. The dissociation constant (Kd) of MFE-23 was shown by fluorescence quench to be 2.5 ± 1.3 nM, indicating the high affinity binding to CEA by comparison with a Kd of 25 nM in the same assay for A5B7, a monoclonal antibody which has produced some of the best colorectal tumour targeting to date [3]. Immunohistochemistry with the purified scFv using a second antibody directed against the myc tag showed a typical CEA-reactive pattern in 20/20 human colorectal adenocarcinomas. The specificity against a range of normal human tissues was examined and the only reactivity was weak and with normal large bowel—this is in contrast to many anti-CEA monoclonal antibodies which commonly show cross reaction with normal lung, spleen, squamous epithelium and neutrophils.

Tumour localisation *in vivo* was studied using LS174T human colorectal tumour xenografts in nude mice and ^{125}Iodine labelled MFE-23. Tissues were removed 24 and 48 h after administration of the radiolabelled MFE-23 and localised radioactivity assessed by gamma counting; four mice were used per group. Results showed $1 \pm 0.3\%$ of the injected activity/g tissue to be localised in the tumour at 24 h and $0.4 \pm 0.1\%$ at 48 h. Due to rapid blood clearance these values gave rise to favourable tumour:blood ratios of 11:1 and 53:1 respectively. Furthermore, on gamma camera imaging of mice given ^{125}Iodine labelled MFE-23 only tumours were visible.

MFE-23 was subsequently purified in accordance with the Cancer Research Campaign operation manual for recombinant clinical products [8] and tested in the clinic. Provisional data on patients shows this scFv to be a superior imaging agent (see Begent *et al.* this meeting) which gives good tumour discrimination at early time points, presumably due to its high affinity for CEA and rapid clearance in accordance with its size. However, the powerful selection system from combinatorial libraries is not limited to this purpose as antibodies with desired characteristics for a wide range of applications may be obtained in the same manner. Antibodies produced using phage technology also have the advantage that their genes are already cloned so genetically engineered antibody derived products such as fusion proteins of antibody with enzymes or toxins can be readily produced. For MFE-23 this has been achieved with various proteins, notably the bacterial enzyme carboxypeptidase G2 which can be used to activate cytotoxic drugs at the tumour site [9].

The ease of isolation and favourable combination of characteristics of MFE-23 illustrate the power of the combinatorial phage library approach in association with a suitable selection system and suggest that this will be used to produce the antibodies of the future.

REFERENCES

1 McCafferty J, Griffiths AD, Winter G, Chiswell DJ. Phage antibodies: filamentous phage displaying antibody variable domains. *Nature* 1990; **348**: 552–4

2 Hawkins RE, Llewelyn MB, Russell SJ. Monoclonal Antibodies in Medicine: Adapting antibodies for clinical use (review). *BMJ* 1992; **305**: 1348–52

3 Lane DM, Eagle KF, Hope-Stone LD, *et al.* Radioimmunotherapy of metastatic colorectal tumours with iodine-131-labelled antibody to carcinoembryonic antigen: phase I/II study with comparative biodistribution of intact and F(ab')$_2$ antibodies. *Br J Cancer* 1994; **70**: 521–5

4 Schlom J, Eggensperger D, Colcher D, *et al.* Therapeutic advantage of high-affinity anticarcinoma radioimmunoconjugates. *Cancer Res* 1992; **52**: 1067–72

5 Hawkins RE, Zhu D, Ovecka M, *et al.* Idiotypic vaccination against B-cell lymphoma. Rescue of variable region gene sequences from biopsy material for assembly as single-chain Fv personal vaccines. *Blood* 1994; **83**: 3279–88

6 Chester KA, Begent RHJ, Robson L, *et al.* A new way to generate clinically useful antibodies. *Lancet* 1994; **343**: 455–6

7 Hawkins RE, Russell SJ, Winter G. Selection of phage antibodies by binding affinity: mimicking affinity maturation. *J Mol Biol* 1992; **226**: 889–96

8 Begent RHJ, Chester KA, Conners T, *et al.* Cancer Research Campaign Operation manual for control recommendations for products derived from recombinant DNA technology prepared for investigational administration to patients with cancer in phase I trials. *Eur J Cancer* 1993; **29A**: 1907–10

9 Bagshawe KD. Towards generating cytotoxic drugs at cancer sites. *Br J Cancer* 1989; **60**: 275–81

Antibody mimics made by molecular imprinting

Klaus Mosbach

Pure and Applied Biochemistry, Chemical Center, University of Lund, Lund, Sweden

PRINCIPLE

The idea of using a specific imprint molecule to coordinate the assembly of synthetic monomers around a molecule of interest, thereby to create a specific host, has been considered and discussed for quite some time. It is only recently, however, that the techniques required have been sufficiently developed to allow realisation of this dream [1]. Two essentially different approaches have been developed—covalent and non-covalent. In both cases, the functional monomers are polymerised in the presence of a print molecule with the functionality in the print molecule interacting with the complementary functionality found in the monomer units. The first approach uses reversible covalent binding of the imprint molecule to the monomer to define the imprint-molecule-monomer interaction, whereas the second approach allows a cocktail of functionalised monomers to 'prearrange' around the imprint molecule by non-covalent interactions (i.e. ionic, hydrophobic, hydrogen bonding, etc.). After completion of polymerisation, the imprint molecule is removed from the polymer, leaving a polymer with recognition sites complementary to the imprint species in both shape and functionality, which has a macroporous structure allowing imprint molecule diffusion into and out of the polymer matrix. This site constitutes an 'induced molecular memory', capable of selectively recognising the imprint species. This technique has become a simple and straightforward method for preparing synthetic polymers of predetermined selectivity. Normally the polymer production technique used has been the bulk polymerisation of the mixture of monomers around the imprint molecules, followed by grinding and extraction of the print species. Particle size is usually in the 25 μm range, suitable for use in a high performance liquid chromatography (HPLC) format.

Over a relatively short period, molecularly imprinted polymers (MIPs) have been developed for a broad range of potential applications. Most of the following examples are taken from work utilising the non-covalent approach, as this seems to be a more direct approach for the application to be discussed, especially those involving chiral separation.

APPLICATIONS

Three main areas of application can be foreseen for the use of MIPs: (1) their use as tailor-made separation materials including antibody binding mimics, (2) their use in enzyme technology and organic synthesis as enzyme mimics or catalytically active polymers, and (3) as sensors in biosensor-like configurations, whereby the polymers are used as substitutes for the biological molecules normally employed.

IMPRINTS AS ANTIBODY MIMICS

Imprints against the bronchodilator drug theophylline and against the tranquilliser diazepam have shown astonishingly specific recognition. In fact, when these MIPs were tested in competitive radioimmuno-style assays, their recognition of related structures was either non-existent or far below that of the original print molecule [2.3]. Amazingly, the cross-reactivity profiles of these MIPs was practically identical to those reported for monoclonal antibodies against these drugs. The anti-theophylline MIPs were used for the determination of theophylline concentrations in patient serum samples, pointing towards their use as stable alternatives to antibodies in

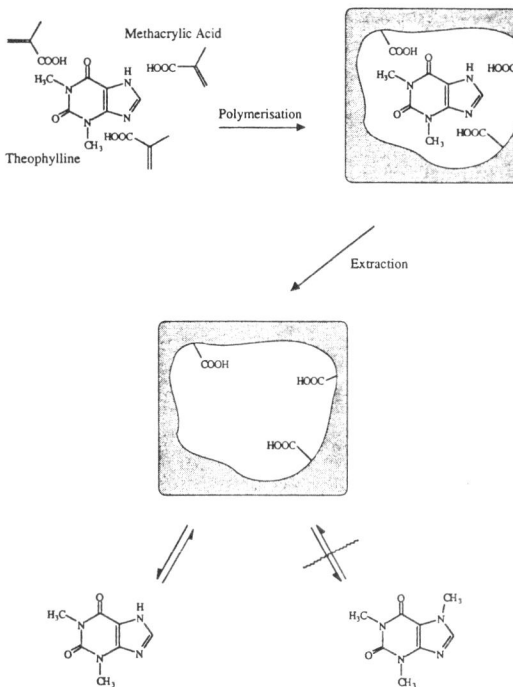

Figure 1. Schematic representation of the preparation of antibody-binding-site mimics. Theophylline, the print molecule, binds effectively to the imprint sites, whereas the structurally closely related caffeine (possessing an additional methyl substituent on the 7-nitrogen which minimises its hydrogen bonding capacity) does not.

conventional immunoassays. The measured Kd constants were in the micromolar range. Some of our more recent studies have involved the successful preparation of imprints against morphine and against leuenkephalin, leading to what could be considered as an artificial opioid receptor. It will be interesting to study and compare molecular recognition in these receptor binding site mimics. Presently we are directing our efforts towards obtaining imprints of compounds against which it is normally difficult to get good antibodies. Thus, we have been able to obtain highly specific molecular imprints against cyclosporin, various macrolide structures, sugars and the pesticide atrazine. We believe that such polymers ('intelligent materials') offer a potentially useful addition to biological antibodies for both immunoassays and in immunoaffinity chromatography due to their robustness, extraordinary stability and ease and cheapness of preparation.

OTHER AREAS OF APPLICATION SUCH AS CHIRAL SEPARATION

The first reported separation of drugs such as β-blockers (aryloxy propanolamines) including (S)-timolol using this technique led to base-line separation [4]. Another drug that was recently separated with this technique into its optical antipodes was (S)naproxen [5].

Of the 500 or so optically active drugs presently on the market, some 90% are administered as racemic mixtures. This fact and the recent requirement by the Food and Drug Administration that for new optically active drugs to be approved, both enantiomers must be treated as separate substances in pharmacokinetic and toxicological profiling, emphasise the demand for improved separation techniques. With all due respect to the current methods for chiral synthesis, enzyme resolution and other techniques for separation of enantiomers including more traditional chiral stationary phases (CSP), more are required. We feel that the technique of molecular imprinting has a great potential in this context as the concept permits one, at least in principle, to obtain specific tailor-made binding polymers for a given separation process. One is thus not confined to the 'trial and error approach' inherent with the different 'old' chiral stationary phases.

REFERENCES

1 Mosbach K. Molecular imprinting. *Trends Biochem Sci* 1994; **19**: 9–14

2 Vlatakis G, Andersson LI, Müller R, Mosbach K. Drug assay using antibody mimics made by molecular imprinting. *Nature* 1993; **361**: 645–7

3 Mosbach K. *US patent* 5.110.833

4 Fischer L, Müller R, Ekberg B, Mosbach K. Direct enantioseparation of β-adrenergic blockers using a chiral stationary phase prepared by molecular imprinting. *J Am Chem Soc* 1991; **113**: 9358–60

5 Kempe M, Mosbach K. Direct resolution of naproxen on a non-covalently molecularly imprinted chiral stationary phase. *J Chromatography A* 1994; **664**: 276–9

Radioimmunotherapy of ovarian cancer in the adjuvant setting

Steve Nicholson
and Agamemnon A. Epenetos
Tumour Targeting Laboratory, Imperial Cancer Research Fund Department of Clinical Oncology, Hammersmith Hospital, Du Cane Road, London, UK

Ovarian cancer accounts for over 4000 deaths per annum in the UK [1]. The majority of patients present with advanced disease, and despite their frequent entry into remission after optimal primary therapy most will relapse and die of their disease: the overall five year survival is around 30%.

Polymorphic epithelial mucin (PEM or epsialin) is a cell-surface glycoprotein which is both aberrantly glycosylated and overexpressed in many adenocarcinomas including those of the breast and ovary. The protein backbone is composed of a variable number of tandem repeats of a peptide of 20 amino acids [2]. Both the carbohydrate side-chains and various epitopes within the peptide are recognised to some extent by the immune system [3,4].

HMFG1 is a murine monoclonal antibody (IgG1) raised against the normal human milk fat globule. Its binding to the PEM on malignant tissue has made it a suitable tool for exploitation in the targeting of radioisotopes. This has been the principal clinical research interest in this laboratory for the past 10 years [5], research which has now led to the initiation of the first phase III clinical trial of radioimmunotherapy in ovarian cancer.

ISOTOPES AND CHELATES

Early work with [131]Iodine-labelled monoclonal antibodies confirmed the feasibility of both intravenous [6] and intraperitoneal administration [7], however the undesired gamma-irradiation of normal tissue limited dose escalation and therefore efficacy. The hope that a pure beta-emitter would more precisely target the delivered radiation has lead to the use of Yttrium-90, which possesses a high-energy beta-particle with a short path length and a relatively short half-life (64 h). Since there is no labelling option analogous to the iodination of tyrosine residues, yttrium radioimmunotherapy requires the introduction of a bifunctional metal chelate capable of being bound to the monoclonal antibody whilst also ligating the metal ion. Dethylene triamine pentaacetic acid (DTPA), the original chelate, is free of any toxicity but is a poor chelator of yttrium. The free ^{90}Y thus released into the circulation is bone-seeking and in our experience caused far greater irradiation of the bone marrow than was predicted to occur from the marrow blood pool. The dose-limiting toxicity was neutropenia and second-step administration of EDTA (ethylene diamine tetraacetic acid) to chelate free yttrium failed to eliminate this sufficiently to allow dose escalation to the desired level [8]. The incorporation of a new macrocyclic chelating agent DOTA ([2-p-nitrobenzyl]-1,4,7,10-tetraazacyclododecane-N,N′,N″,N‴-tetraacetic acid) allowed more stable chelation, but the rigid cyclic structure was found to be profoundly immunogenic, causing rashes universally and additional problems such as arthritis, neuropathy and presumed serum-sickness [9]. The non-macrocyclic bifunctional chelate CITC-DTPA (isothiocyanatobenzyl-DTPA) was chosen as a potential for conjugation due to a less rigid—and therefore less immunogenic—cyclic structure which is nevertheless a strong chelator of the ^{90}Y [10]. A phase I-II study (see below) has confirmed tolerable immunogenicity while

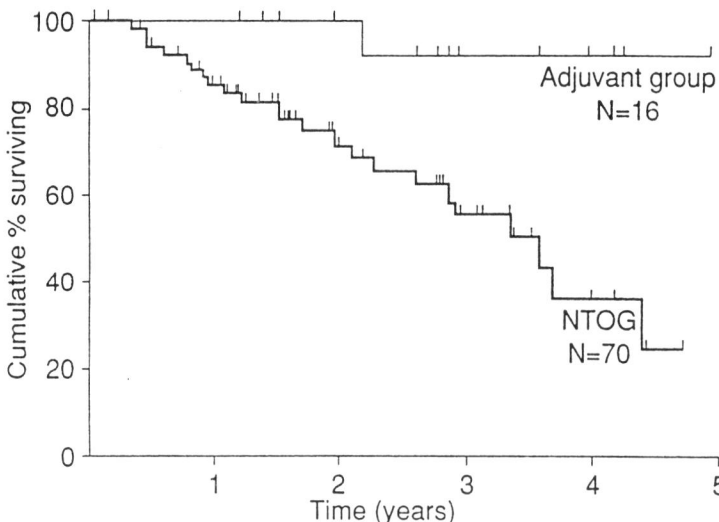

Figure 1.   Survival from evaluation at end of primary treatment (NTOG=North Thames Ovary Group)

allowing escalation to a delivered activity of 34 mCi in a single intraperitoneal dose [11].

It has been estimated that an untargeted dose of 45–50 Gy [12] to the peritoneum is required to sterilise residual tumour following debulking surgery and chemotherapy. Stewart *et al.* have shown, however, that the radiation dose to the serosa equates to 21.7 cGy per mCi of isotope [13], and that the total dose received by the peritoneum is less than 5 Gy [14]. It has also been stated, however, that conventional dosimetry is probably inappropriate when applied to radioimmunotherapy [15].

PHASE I-II TRIAL

Fifty-two patients with disease stages Ia to IV received intraperitoneal radioimmunotherapy as a single dose of ^{90}Y-conjugate-HMFG1 of known activity made up to a total antibody dose of 25 mg with unlabelled HMFG1 and infused in 1.5 litres of Hartman's solution. Treatment was administered after a laparoscopy to assess disease status and to ensure that excessive adhesions would not hinder the free flow of the infusion. Disease status ranged from bulky intraperitoneal masses to complete remission (under which circumstance the patient was considered to have been treated in the adjuvant setting).

All patients developed human anti-mouse antibodies (HAMA), and those patients who received DOTA or CITC-

DTPA as the chelate developed anti-chelate antibodies [16]. Median survival for the patients with residual disease was only 11 months, however those patients treated in the adjuvant setting (stages Ic to IV) showed enhanced survival. Figure 1 shows the actuarial survival curve of a subgroup of adjuvantly-treated patients, who had stages IIb and above, compared with that of the patients in the North Thames Ovarian Group study, which examined survival in patients with similar disease stages following negative second-look laparoscopy [17]. This comparison suffers from the small sample size for radioimmunotherapy patients and from their relatively early stage of follow-up. More prolonged follow-up seems to confirm a survival advantage for this group (unpublished).

DISCUSSION

The dose of radiation being considered insufficient to account for a cytotoxic effect, this raises the question of the mechanism of action of this treatment. The theory of idiotypic networks [18] has been proven in patients receiving monoclonal antibody therapy [19], as has T-cell memory in patients undergoing radioimmunotherapy [20]. It is possible that ^{90}Y-HMFG1 is acting as an idiotypic vaccine, in which case the intrinsic immunogenicity of a murine antibody may confer advantages over the use of a human or humanised monoclonal antibody. This scenario would imply that the bifunctional chelate is acting as a vaccine adjuvant, a theory supported by the generation of anti-chelate antibodies and the immunological 'fall-out' (rashes, arthritides, neuropathy, serum-sickness) seen in these patients.

A phase III trial has now begun, aiming to confirm or refute the above findings; all eligible patients who consent to participate will undergo laparoscopy and peritoneal lavage for cytology. If complete remission is confirmed patients receive either intraperitoneal radioimmunotherapy (activity 18 mCi/m^2) or no further treatment. Inclusion criteria are stages Ic to IV, clinical and radiological complete remission after platinum-based chemotherapy, and normal CA125. The primary end-point is survival and patients are also assessed for quality of life and immunological response to treatment. This trial is being funded by the Imperial Cancer Research Fund, who have been the sponsors for all the work conducted in this laboratory.

REFERENCES

1 Austoker J. Cancer prevention in primary care. *BMJ* 1994; **309**: 315–20

2 Taylor-Papadimitriou J, Stewart L, Burchell J, Beverley P. The polymorphic epithelial mucin as a target for immunotherapy. *Ann N Y Acad Sci* 1993; **690**: 69–79

3 Kotera Y, Fontenot JD, Pecher G, Metzgar RS, Finn OJ. Humoral immunity against a tandem repeat epitope of human mucin MUC1 in sera from breast, pancreatic, and colon cancer patients. *Cancer Res* 1994; **54**: 2856–60

4 Jerome KR, Barnd DL, Bendt KM *et al*. Cytotoxic T-lymphocytes derived from patients with breast adenocarcinoma recognize an epitope present on the protein core of a mucin molecule preferentially expressed by malignant cells. *Cancer Res* 1991; **51**: 2908–16

5 Epenetos AA. Hammersmith Hospital Oncology Group, Imperial Cancer Research Fund. Antibody-guided irradiation of malignant lesions: three cases illustrating a new method of treatment. *Lancet* 1984; **2**: 1441–3

6 DeNardo SJ, DeNardo GL, O'Grady LF, *et al*. Treatment of B-cell malignancies with ^{131}I-Lym-1 monoclonal antibodies. *Int J Cancer* 1988; **suppl 3**: 96–101

7 Epenetos AA, Munro AJ, Stewart JSW, *et al*. Antibody-guided irradiation of advanced ovarian cancer with intraperitoneally administered radiolabelled monoclonal antibodies. *J Clin Oncol* 1987; **5**: 1890–9

8 Stewart JSW, Hird V, Snook D, *et al*. Intraperitoneal yttrium-90-labelled monoclonal antibody in ovarian cancer. *J Clin Oncol* 1990; **8**: 1941–50

9 Kosmas C, Snook D, Gooden CS, *et al*. Development of humoral immune responses against a macrocyclic chelating agent (DOTA) in cancer patients receiving radioimmunoconjugates for imaging and therapy. *Cancer Res* 1992; **52**: 904–11

10 Maraveyas A, Snook D, Hird V, *et al*. Pharmacokinetics and toxicity of an Yttrium-90-CITC-DTPA-HMFG1 radioimmunoconjugate for intraperitoneal radioimmunotherapy of ovarian cancer. *Cancer* 1994; **73 (suppl)**: 1067–75

11 Hird V, Maraveyas A, Snook D, *et al*. Adjuvant therapy of ovarian cancer with radioactive monoclonal antibody. *Br J Cancer* 1993; **68**: 403–6

12 Dembo AJ. Abdominopelvic radiotherapy in ovarian cancer: a 10-year experience. *Cancer* 1985; **55**: 2285–90

13 Stewart JSW, Hird V, Snook D, Sullivan M, Myers MJ, Epenetos AA. Intraperitoneal ^{131}I- and ^{90}Y-labelled monoclonal antibodies for ovarian cancer: Pharmacokinetics and normal tissue dosimetry. *Int J Cancer* 1988; **suppl 3**: 71–6

14 Stewart JS, Hird V, Sullivan M, Snook D, Epenetos AA. Intraperitoneal radioimmunotherapy for ovarian cancer. *Br J Obstet Gynaecol* 1989; **96**: 529–36

15 Myers MJ. Dosimetry for radiolabelled antibodies—macro or micro. *Int J Cancer* 1988; **suppl 2**: 71–3

16 Kosmas C, Maraveyas A, Gooden CS, Snook D, Meares CF, Epenetos AA. Co-ordinate elevation of anti-chelate antibodies after intraperitoneal administration of stable yttrium-90-labelled monoclonal antibody immunoconjugates for ovarian cancer therapy. *Cancer* (1994)

17 Lambert HE, Rustin GJS, Gregory WM, Nelstrop AE. A randomised trial comparing single-agent carboplatin with carboplatin followed by radiotherapy for advanced ovarian cancer; a North Thames Ovary Group study. *J Clin Oncol* 1993; **11**: 440–8

18 Jerne NK. Towards a network theory of the immune system. *Ann Immunol* 1974; **125C**: 373–89

19 Courtenay-Luck NS, Epenetos AA, Sivolapenko GB, Larche M, Barkans JR, Ritter MA. Development of anti-idiotypic antibodies against tumour antigens and autoantigens in ovarian cancer patients treated intraperitoneally with mouse monoclonal antibodies. *Lancet* 1988; **ii**: 894–6

20 Kosmas C, Epentos AA, Courtenay-Luck NS. Patients receiving murine monoclonal antibody therapy for malignancy develop T cells that proliferate *in vitro* in response to these antibodies as antigens. *Br J Cancer* 1991; **64**: 494–500

Intralesional therapy of glioma

P. Riva[1], A. Arista[2], C. Sturiale[2], S. Lazzari[3], G. Franceschi[1], G. Moscatelli[1], G. Sarti[3], F. Campori[1], N. Riva[1], M. Casi[1], R. Gentile[1]

[1]Nuclear Medicine Deptartment and Istituto Oncologico Romagnolo; [2]Neurosurgery Department and [3]Medical Physic Department "M. Bufalini" Hospital, Cesena, Italy

INTRODUCTION

Radioimmunotherapy (RIT) of solid tumours can be successfully applied when large amounts of radiolabelled monoclonal antibodies (MoAbs) are concentrated in target tissue for a long time, so intensifying the irradiation [1]. Since intravenous administration does not lead to sufficient accretion of the antibodies on the tumour, loco-regional routes of injections such as intrapleural, intraperitoneal, and intrathecal [2–4] were utilised aiming to enhance MoAbs uptake in target neoplastic tissue. With the same aim, the intralesional [5,6] route was chosen in 53 patients with malignant glioma (52 of the brain and one of the spinal cord). In fact this tumour presents an anatomical and clinical behaviour suitable for this approach. It usually does not diffuse outside the brain but spreads covertly around the primary lesion. Complete recovery is possible following intratumoural administration of a therapeutic agent. The intratumoural injection is quite a difficult and time-consuming technique. But it represents, so far, the best method to overcome the limits encountered when monoclonal antibodies are administered intravenously: low concentration of antibodies in the tumour, high background radioactivity and non-specific uptake in normal organs such as liver, spleen, kidney and bone marrow.

MATERIALS AND METHOD

Two murine IgG1 monoclonal antibodies BC-2 and BC-4 (SORIN-BIOMEDICA, Italy) have been utilised singly or as a cocktail. They react strongly with tenascin which is an extracellular antigen found in impressive amounts in the stroma both of the core and the periphery of malignant glioma. By contrast it is totally absent in normal cerebral tissue [7]. This histological feature is very favourable for RIT applications. In fact malignant cells are surrounded on all sides by large numbers of tenascin antigens and are easily reached by isotope beta rays conjugated with antitenascin antibodies, since they lie very close to extracellular antigens. By this means almost all neoplastic elements are hit and damaged by radiations. Conversely the antigens present on cell membrane are expressed less abundantly and less homogeneously, allowing less satisfactory tumour targeting. The MoAbs were labelled with ^{131}I whose dose per cycle was progressively increased according to an escalating schedule (5,15,25,30,40,50 60,70 mCi). The maximum cumulative ^{131}I dose was given to a patient who underwent six cycles and consisted of 212 mCi.

Patients

Fifty-three patients have so far undergone intralesional RIT: 47 of these are evaluable—since four died of cardiovascular disease and the remaining two received RIT only a few months ago. The patients can be subdivided in two subsets: a) 27 patients suffering a relapse which developed on average 6–8 months after the treatment of primary tumour. Twenty-four of them underwent further operation but only in 12 cases did surgery obtain a total or subtotal removal of neoplastic tissue. b) Twenty cases with newly diagnosed malignant gliomas who received treatment

Table 1.   Features of the patients

	Patients	Further surgery	Bulky residual	Minimal disease
Primary tumour	20	//	6	14
Recurrent disease	27	24	15	12

following surgery and external radiotherapy of primary tumour. In 14 out of 20 previous cases therapy succeeded in statisfactory debulking and patients received RIT when the disease was minimal or microscopic (Table 1). To summarise, we recruited 21 patients with bulky lesions (15 recurrent and 6 primary) while 26 cases presented a very reduced or minimal remnant (12 recurrent and 14 primary). Direct intratumour RIT was given by using a removable (15 cases) or indwelling catheter (38 patients). In most patients multiple courses were carried out either when the persistence of disease was radiologically demonstrated to destroy residual glioma tissue or in order to consolidate the response even if the CT scan did not give any evidence of tumour. Second and third treatments were given within 1–2 months. Then further applications were performed at 3–6 month intervals, depending on the clinical and radiological course of disease. Altogether 129 courses were performed. Many patients had three or four cycles, two received five and one case six treatments. The radio-immunotherapy protocol was stopped when either clinical data and CT scan, MRI and brain SPECT with Tc99m DTPA has shown completely normal results for at least six months.

RESULTS

a) Adverse effects

Radioimmunotherapy applications did not produce any systemic, haematological, hepatic or renal side effects. In some patients a transitory headache was recorded. In three cases a meningismus which lasted no more than 24 h was observed. It was due to a diffusion of MoAbs' proteins into the CSF owing to communications between the tumour and cerebral ventricles or cisternae. The administration of steroids and NSAIDs led to complete recovery of the patients within 24 h. No signs of late brain damage were encountered such as memory loss, decrease of attention, and of learning, vision reduction, dyssomnia and so on. Forty-five per cent of cases developed human antimouse

antibody (HAMA) [8] whose mean titre was 1/46, and ranged between 1/1 to 1/1024. Nevertheless HAMA presence did not give rise to clinical complications nor did it change the biodistribution of MAbs during subsequent RIT courses.

Biokinetics and dosimetry

The biodistribution of radiopharmaceuticals following intralesional injection proved to be very effective, producing an intense and selective irradiation of glioma mass. The average percentage of injected dose concentrated per gram of tumour was quite high—4.9% (at 24 h)—and did not decrease during the course of subsequent administrations. The duration of residence time of antibodies in the neoplastic tissue was very prolonged. Their effective half-life on average was 53 h and this value remained stable in further RIT applications. In many patients an immunoscintigraphy carried out 40–65 days after the injection demonstrated a persistent uptake of radiolabelled MoAbs only in the site of disease, completely sparing both normal cerebral tissue and healthy organs. The dosimetry data, evaluated by means of both MIRD and Monte Carlo [9,10] formulae, proved the ability of the intralesional approach to deliver a very high dose to malignant gliomas. The radiation to the tumour was on average more than 30.000 cGy even during repeated administrations. In patients who had two or more RIT cycles the cumulative dose was remarkably increased exceeding, when four or five courses were carried out, 150.000 cGy. By contrast liver, kidneys and bone marrow received very low doses (<150 cGy). The dose to the thyroid was moderate enough (<400 cGy) to preserve its endocrine function. At the same time the irradiation of glioma was rather homogeneous owing to the diffuse spread of MoAbs from the site of injection through the total neoplastic tissue, assessed both by sequential scintigraphies and, when possible, by autoradiography. One patient who had already undergone two RIT courses,was given a tracer dose before further surgery which was necessary owing to tumour relapse. The autoradiography of the resected specimen demonstrated a complete and homogeneous spread of specific MAb only into a small area of viable neoplastic tissue but not in a near large necrotic area produced by previous RIT. Moreover the specific targeting was proved in one case who was injected firstly with an irrelevant antibody and, a week later,with the specific BC-2 MoAb. In this case the uptake of specific antibody and its residence time in the tumour was

Table 2.   Objective response

	No. patients	Duration (months)
Progression	20	5.6
Stable disease	9	9.4
Partial remission	7	9.5
Complete remission	11	18

considerably higher than was recorded when the irrelevant immunoglobulin was employed.

Clinical response

The clinical effects of intralesional RIT have to be considered rather promising. The treatment significantly prolonged the patients' life span. The median survival of our group is, at present, 18 months versus 12 months achievable by means of current treatments [11]. Moreover quality of life was significantly improved. The objective response (Table 2) showed 20 cases of progressive disease, nine tumour stabilisations (median duration 9.4 months), seven partial remissions (median 9.5 months) and 11 complete remissions (median 18 months, range 4–50). The response rate (RR) was 38.3%, a result never previously obtained by means of surgery and radiotherapy alone. Nineteen patients are alive at 14 months (median) after RIT. Nine patients are still alive and free of disease at 16 months (median). Analysing the factors which could affect the response to RIT, we found that the determining factor of positive response to RIT is the small volume of the disease. In patients with a macroscopic lesion, the response rate was 23.8%. By contrast, when the disease was reduced, the response rate was 46.1%. In this group best results were obtained in patients who had radioimmunotherapy after the traditional treatments of primary tumour (response rate 60%). In recurrent lesions the response rate was 50%. Nine patients underwent further surgical operation following one or more courses of intralesional RIT. In all cases large areas of necrosis and fibrosis produced by previous treatment were observed. In the group of 29 patients in whom the tumour relapsed in spite of RIT applications we observed that in 17 (58.6%) cases the neoplastic recurrence occurred in tumour bed but in the remaining 12 patients (41.4%) it was outside the primary lesion. So, in these cases RIT succeeded in sterilising most neoplastic cells placed in the site of primary

glioma but did not reach the tumour clusters in more distant areas. Moreover the regrowth of tumour in its bed, where RIT should have produced maximum effect, was recorded in the majority of cases in the group with bulky neoplastic lesions. In this pathological situation the antibodies cannot target all neoplastic elements since they are often well sheltered.

Conclusions

The intralesional radioimmunotherapy of gliomas proved to be a procedure well tolerated by patients and did not give rise to early or late side effects. In particular the normal cerebral tissue did not present any early or late alteration following the local administration of quite large quantities both of antibody and ^{131}I. The loco-regional administration of radiopharmaceutical agents, therefore, enables the accumulation of a high level of radioactivity in the neoplastic tissue, for a long time. So the radiation dose delivered to the target tumour was impressively higher than the dose achievable by means of external radiotherapy. As a consequence the clinical response was definitively better than the outcomes so far obtained even when combining surgery, radiotherapy and chemotherapy. The quality of life is proved and the life expectancy was significantly lengthened compared with cases submitted to conventional treatment. Moreover many patients (11/47) experienced a complete and long lasting remission of the tumour. The best approach to giving intralesional RIT is to perform this treatment soon after the conventional treatment (surgery, radiotherapy and, in particular cases, chemotherapy) of the primary lesion, especially if the remaining disease is minimal or microscopic, as an adjuvant. The use of Y-90 [12], which is a stronger beta emitter with respect to ^{131}I, could lead to damage and destruction of the neoplastic cell clusters outside the lesion which, if spared by RIT carried out with ^{131}I, can give rise to tumour relapse.

Acknowledgment

This work was supported by the National Research Council program (Italy): Clinical Applications of Oncology Research, subproject 8.

REFERENCES

1 Goldenberg DM, Griffith GL. Radioimmunotherapy of cancer: arming the missiles. *J Nucl Med* 1992; **33**: 1110–12

2 Hird V, Snook C, Kosmas C, *et al*. Intraperitoneal Radioimmunotherapy with yttrium-90 labelled immuno-conjugates. In: Epenetos A, ed. *Monoclonal antibodies: applications in clinical oncology*. London: Chapman and Hall Medical, 1991; 267–71

3 Pectasides D, Steward S, Curtenay-Luck N, *et al*. Antibody-guided irradiation of malignant pleural and pericardial effusions. *Br J Cancer* 1986; **53**: 727–32

4 Benjamin JC, Moss T, Moseley RP, Maxwell R, Coakham HB. Cerebral distribution of immunoconjugate after treatment for neoplastic meningitis using an intrathecal radiolabeled monoclonal antibody. *Neurosurgery* 1989; **24**: 253–8

5 Riva P, Arista A, Sturiale C, *et al*. Treatment of intracranial human glioblastoma by direct intratumoral administration of I-131 labelled antitenascin monoclonal antibody BC-2. *Int J Cancer* 1992; **51**: 7–13

6 Riva P, Arista A, Tison V, *et al*. Intralesional radioimmunotherapy of malignant glioma: an effective treatment in recurrent tumors. *Cancer* 1994; **73** (suppl): 1076–82

7 Natali PG, Zardi L. Tenascin: an exameric adhesive glycoprotein. *Int J Cancer* 1989; **4** (suppl): 66–8

8 Dillman RO. Human antimouse and antiglobulin responses to monoclonal antibodies. *Antibody Immunoconj Radiopharm* 1990; **3**: 1–8

9 MIRD Pamphlet, No 11. NY: Society of Nuclear Medicine, 1985

10 Loevinger R, Berman M. A scheme for absorbed dose calculation for biologically distributed radionuclides. MIRD pamphlet no. 1. *J Nucl Med* 1968; **9** (suppl. 1): 7

11 Chang CH, Horton J, Schoenfeld D, *et al*. Comparison of postoperative radiotherapy and combined postoperative radiotherapy and chemotherapy in the multidisciplinary management of malignant gliomas. *Cancer* 1983; **52**: 997–1007

12 Hnatowich DJ, Mardirossian G, Rose PG, *et al*. Intraperitoneal therapy of ovarian cancer with Yttrium-90-labeled monoclonal antibodies: preliminary observations. *Antibody, Immunoconj Radiopharm* 1991; **4**: 359–72.

Therapy of meningeal tumours

John T. Kemshead, Kirsten I. Hopkins,
Christopher L. Chandler
*The Imperial Cancer Research Fund, Paediatric &
Neuro-Oncology Group, Frenchay Hospital, Bristol, UK*

Fifty-four patients with a variety of malignancies have been recruited to this study, which entails targeting ^{131}I-monoclonal antibodies (MoAbs) to tumour cells within the cerebrospinal fluid (CSF) and the meninges. Patients were eligible for entry into the study if they had imageable disease observed by either CT or MRI scan and/or free-floating malignant cells in the CSF. Individuals were excluded if they were considered to have bulky solid tumour deposits (>1 cm diameter), had received either recent chemotherapy or external beam radiotherapy, or were judged to have a life expectancy of less than three months. After piloting this approach to treatment for a variety of different malignancies, our research work has concentrated on patients with either primitive neuroectodermal tumours (PNETs) or those with isolated central nervous system (CNS) leukaemia. In the PNET group, 15 patients were under 21 and 11 were adults, whereas eight out of nine treated for CNS leukaemia/lymphoma were under the age of 18.

Antibodies where chosen depending upon their binding to individual patient's tumour. MoAb M340 was used for the majority of the PNET patients (18/26), whilst either anti-CD10 and/or CD19 MoAbs were chosen for the leukaemia/lymphoma patients. All reagents were prepared to clinical grade, with extensive testing both before and after conjugation of the radio label to ensure bio-reactivity, sterility, lack of pyrogenecity and the absence of aggregates. Prior to administration of radioimmunoconjugate, patients were placed on a regimen to block uptake of ^{131}I into their thyroid, and in the majority of cases they were also given phenytoin and dexamethasone. MoAbs were injected via an Ommaya reservoir leading into one of the cerebral ventricles. A few individuals had ventriculo-peritoneal shunts. These were clipped off before the injection of ^{131}I-MoAb.

In the PNET group, 15 patients received a single injection of immunoconjugate, eight received two and three received three injections. Five of the leukaemic patients received a single injection of ^{131}I-MoAb, two received two injections and two received three injections spaced four to six weeks apart, unless myelosuppression prevented this timing. Marked dose escalation was attempted when patients had repeated injections of immunoconjugate. This was possible as pharmacokinetic studies revealed that the anti-mouse Ig response generated after the first injection of MoAb was far greater in the blood compartment than in the CSF. Consequently, blood clearance of the conjugate was more rapid following repeated injections of ^{131}I-MoAb, whilst clearance from the CSF remained relatively unchanged.

Although the study was not co-ordinated in a formal Phase I dose escalation fashion, the injected activity given for the first injection of immunoconjugate was increased from 555 to 2588 MBq over the period of the study. Acute toxicity varied markedly between patients. Within the PNET and leukaemic patient groups no toxicity was observed in 13, whilst a self-limiting aseptic meningitis was noted in 20, lasting up to 48 h from antibody administration. In one individual, a progressive bulbar palsy was observed and the patient needed aspiration before gradually recovering. A second patient went into status epilepticus. This latter incident may not have been directly related to the therapy, as the patient had a history of fits prior to treatment.

The medium term and dose limiting toxicity of this approach to the treatment of diffuse disease within the CSF pathways is myelosuppression. This is caused by the passage of radioimmunoconjugate from the CSF to the blood compartment. Peak blood levels of conjugate reach 30–40% of the injected dose approximately 24–48 h after antibody administration. Myelotoxicity was unpredictable and in total occurred in nine individuals. This appeared to be related more to the degree of prior therapy patients had been given rather than to the dose of immunoconjugate received. Apart from one individual, all patients suffering myelotoxicity received over 1850 MBq of ^{131}I-MoAb. The exception was a leukaemic patient who developed myelotoxicity after receiving only 1610 MBq of immunoconjugate, but he was kept on maintenance chemotherapy during the antibody treatment. Myelotoxicity was, however, not seen in all individuals receiving high doses of ^{131}I-MoAb (<1800 MBq) and has not been observed in any patient receiving their second or third injections of up to 5,500 MBq of conjugate. No medium term neurological damage has been noted in any of the patients receiving ^{131}I-MoAb injected into the CSF.

Despite the small numbers of patients investigated, and the difficulties associated with accurately defining response criteria, an attempt has been made to determine the effectiveness of targeted therapy. This clearly differed between the PNET and leukaemic patients. In the PNET group, complete disappearance of disease was observed in five patients, with remissions ranging from three to 63 months, whilst a partial response was noted in six. In the latter individuals, this took the form of clearance of cells from the CSF whilst imageable tumour deposits appeared relatively unchanged. Static disease was noted in three individuals and no response recorded in eight. Four patients were not evaluable for response due to a variety of complicating factors. In the leukaemic group, no response was observed in one individual, but in the other seven complete clearance of cells from the CSF was recorded for relatively short periods ranging from six to 16 weeks. One patient was not evaluable for response due to his receiving chemotherapy along with ^{131}I-MoAb.

From the detailed pharmacokinetic measurements taken on the clearance of immunoconjugate from the ventricular CSF and blood, mathematical models have been established to predict the dose to ventricular CSF, subarachnoid CSF, ventricular wall, whole brain, bone marrow and whole body (Table 1). Space does not permit a detailed description as to how these estimates were derived, but these models are described elsewhere [1]. Whilst it is possible to approximate dose to tumour cells within the CSF, as this is equivalent to that received by the CSF itself, calculation of dose to tumour lining the meninges is not possible. This depends upon variables such as the degree of MoAb binding and the degree of diffusion of conjugate into the tumour deposits; data which is not easily obtained.

The above dosimetric calculations point to the advantages that may be obtained by targeting radionuclides and also indicate how this approach to therapy may be improved. Firstly, clearance of immunoconjugate from the ventricular CSF approximates that of the half life of the CSF within the ventricles. This means that the level of immunoconjugate and consequently the dose rate to the ventricular CSF and the surrounding wall falls rapidly. It may be possible to maintain the dose rate at a higher level for a longer period of time by splitting the injection of conjugate into three, given some 8 h apart. This fractionation is independent of the benefit that may be achieved by repeating administration of the immunoconjugate at four to six-week intervals.

Another major advantage that may be gained from targeting is to use cocktails of MoAbs. Antibodies are being radiolabelled to a maximum specific activity where antigen binding is not inhibited. Dose escalation results in more isotope being given, but also the level of MoAb administered is also increased. In a situation of minimal residual disease, this results in gross antibody excess over

Table 1. Doses to organs and tissues surrounding the CSF following administration of ^{131}I-MoAbs to the lateral ventricles

	Mean (Gy)	Range (Gy)	Mean/MBq administered (Gy)
Whole body	0.25	0.093–0.7	1.4×10^{-4}
Bone marrow	1.58	0.15–2.84	0.93×10^{-3}
Ventricular CSF	54	14–92	3.1×10^{-2}
Subarachnoid CSF	35.3	13.1–81	1.96×10^{-2}
Ventricular wall	9.9	1.8–18.6	5.7×10^{-3}
Subarachnoid wall	6.67	1.25–13.21	3.6×10^{-3}
Normal brain	0.8	0.22–1.4	4.5×10^{-4}

available antigen. Consequently, the vast majority of dose deposition to tumour is brought about by a non-targeted element. This contradicts the whole philosophy behind antibody targeting and suggests that similar results could be obtained through the use of an irrelevant radiolabelled protein used as a carrier to hold the isotope in the CSF compartment for as long as possible. The use of cocktails of MoAbs would increase the number of antigens available for targeting, potentially maximising the time that the isotope remains within the CSF compartment. This would, therefore, increase both the dose and dose rate given to the malignant population. *In vitro* data using a panel of anti-leukaemic MoAbs supports this hypothesis. Currently, we are attempting to produce further MoAbs of appropriate specificity to target to PNETs within the CSF and in addition explore the potential of using alternative approaches to enhance binding of radiolabelled MoAb to the surface of a relatively limited number of tumour cells

REFERENCE

1 Papanastassiou V, Pizer BL, Chandler CL, Zananiri TF, Kemshead JT, Hopkins KI. Pharmacokinetics and dose estimates following intrathecal administration of 131I-MoAbs for the treatment of CNS malignancies. *Int J Rad Oncol Biol Physics* (1994) (in press).

Radiolabelled antibody therapy of relapsed B-cell lymphomas

Oliver W. Press

Departments of Medicine and Biological Structure, University of Washington, and the Fred Hutchinson Cancer Research Center, Seattle, WA, USA

Over the past decade, our group in Seattle has conducted a series of investigations to determine the utility of treating patients with relapsed B-cell lymphomas with either unmodified monoclonal antibodies or radiolabelled antibodies. An initial study employing intravenous administration of an unmodified anti-CD20 antibody (1F5) demonstrated that circulating B-cells were rapidly eliminated from the bloodstream, and that transient lymph node regressions occurred in two of four patients. Unfortunately, these patients rapidly relapsed with recurrent lymphoma after intervals of 10 days to six weeks. Consequently, we endeavoured to enhance the potency and durability of antibody therapy by conjugating ^{131}I to a series of anti-B-cell monoclonal antibodies targeting CD20 (B1, 1F5), CD37 (MB-1), DR (anti-LYM1), or surface idiotype.

In a phase I dose escalation trial, patients were assessed on successive weeks with 0.5, 2.5, or 10 mg/kg of antibody trace-labelled with 5–10 mCi of ^{131}I and assessed by serial gamma camera imaging, tumour biopsies, and computed tomography. Absorbed radiation doses to tumour sites and normal organs were estimated using the MIRD method.

In 24 of the 43 patients on the study, every assessable tumour was estimated to receive more radiation than any of the normal organs (except the thyroid gland) and this circumstance was defined as a 'favourable biodistribution'.

Nineteen patients with 'favourable' biodistributions were given high dose radioimmunotherapy with 280–777 mCi of ^{131}I-labelled antibodies according to a dose escalation scheme delivering <1000, <1500, <1675, <2025, <2375, <2725, and <3075 cGy to normal organs to in cohorts of 3 patients each. Moderate nausea was the only significant acute toxicity.

Myelosuppression requiring reinfusion of autologous, purged marrow occurred 2–4 weeks following treatment in 15 patients. Two patients developed severe, but reversible cardiopulmonary toxicity (after absorbed lung doses of 2725 and 3075 cGy), resulting in termination of the Phase I study with a presumed maximal tolerated dose (MTD) of approximately 2700 cGy to the lungs and heart. Sixteen of the 19 treated patients achieved complete remissions, two had partial responses, and nine patients had a minor response. The mean response duration is >21 months. Nine patients remain in continuous complete remission after 20+ to 71+ months.

A subsequent phase II study is being conducted at the maximally tolerated dose of ^{131}I-B1 determined in the Phase I study. To date, 24 patients have been entered onto this study, 21 have achieved therapeutic infusions of ^{131}I-B1 (345–785 mCi). Eighteen patients have sufficient follow-up to evaluate for responses, and 12 complete remissions have been achieved so far. Three additional patients have progressively shrinking tumours, but have not yet achieved complete tumour disappearance. All patients experienced myelosuppression and underwent autologous bone marrow reinfusion. Seven of 20 had grade 2–3 nausea, and one patient developed fatal *Escherichia coli* septic shock while neutropenic. Further observation will be necessary to determine the durability of the remissions induced with ^{131}I therapy, but preliminary results suggest that long term remissions can be routinely obtained with less toxicity than conventional bone marrow transplant conditioning regimens.

Antibody targeted therapy of colorectal cancer

Richard Begent

Cancer Research Campaign Targeting and Imaging Group, Royal Free Hospital School of Medicine, London, UK

INTRODUCTION

Colorectal cancer is the second commonest cause of death from cancer in the United Kingdom; approximately 65% of the people who develop the condition die from it, usually as a result of metastatic disease. There is, therefore, an urgent need for effective systemic therapy and antibody targeted therapy provides one of the most promising new approaches.

The therapy is based on antibody targeting to antigens expressed selectively by colorectal carcinoma. One of the most promising targets is carcinoembryonic antigen (CEA), which is present in all colorectal tumours, and on average in about 80% of cells within the tumour. There is however, wide variation between individuals in the extent of CEA expression and in tumour localisation [1]. Other antibodies used in targeting colorectal cancer include 17-1A and A33 which are directed against different cell surface antigens. These antigens are also expressed in lesser concentrations on the luminal surface of normal colonic mucosa. Selective therapy depends on this mucosally expressed antigen being inaccessible to antibodies and experimental data suggest that the tight junctions between gastrointestinal epithelial cells do indeed deny access of circulating IgG antibodies to the luminal surface of the intestine.

EXPERIMENTAL MODELS

Experimental tumour models of human colon carcinoma grown as xenografts in nude mice have been used to investigate different therapeutic approaches. These studies have principally used radiolabelled antibodies (radioimmunotherapy) and antibody directed enzyme prodrug therapy (ADEPT). The latter is dealt with separately at this conference. The ratio between tumour and normal tissues can be enhanced by using a clearance system to remove antitumour antibody from the circulation without correspondingly removing it from the circulation. This can be achieved with a second antibody directed against the antitumour antibody [2] or by biotinylating the antitumour antibody and administering streptavidin to complex circulating antibody molecules thus accelerating their clearance [3].

Antibodies radiolabelled with beta-emitting radionuclides ^{131}Iodine(^{131}I) or yttrium^{90} (^{90}Y) have been used and compared with antibodies with no specificity for colon carcinoma. These show a therapeutic effect which is specific to the antitumour antibody and in some cases established tumours can be eradicated [4]. The animal model system has provided a basis for testing potential improvements in therapy.

CLINICAL RADIOIMMUNOTHERAPY

Clinical studies have been principally with antitumour antibodies radiolabelled with ^{131}I. Clinical investigations of targeted therapy is greatly assisted by assessment of the distribution of antibody in tumour and normal tissue serially after administration. This can be achieved with ^{131}I using a gamma camera which images the gamma emission of ^{131}I to determine antibody distribution [5,6]. Single photon emission tomography is used with correction for Compton scatter and attenuation to produce an estimate of the concentration of radioactivity in a chosen volume of tumour and normal tissues. Repeated studies after administration of radiolabelled antibody can be used to show the cumulative radiation dose, dose rate at any time point and rate of clearance from each tissue. Different antibody preparations and different individuals can be compared in order to understand antibody targeting and improve therapy.

The resulting studies show that with intact IgG antibodies the highest concentrations in the tumour is achieved after 24–48 h and that values in the tumour normally exceed those in blood and normal tissues by this time. Clearance from the tumour is slower than from normal tissues [7]. The effectiveness of radioimmunotherapy depends on cumulative radiation dose and maximum dose rate. The toxicity is principally the result of bone marrow suppression and is related to radiation dose in the blood which irradiates the marrow during circulation.

The best ratios of cumulative radiation dose in tumour and blood are approximately 4:1 and there is great variation between patients; and in some cases the ratio may be no more than 1:1. It is estimated that bone marrow receives one-third the radiation dose of blood and therefore these ratios may reasonably be multiplied by three in favour of the tumour giving a range of 3:1 to 12:1 in favour of tumour.

The maximum dose rates are important as there is a theoretical threshold which must be exceeded before tumour cells are killed faster than they grow. This is particularly relevant in antibody-targeted therapy because the radiation is given over several days which means that the maximum rate is much lower than for external beam radiotherapy.

Responses have been seen in patients receiving maximum dose rates between 1 and 6 cGy per hour, but overall about 10% of patients have responses to ^{131}I antibody directed against CEA. Whilst this is an encouraging start there is a need to improve the technology and particularly to increase maximum dose rate.

IMPROVING ANTIBODY TARGETING

Vascular manipulation

One approach to this is to manipulate tumour blood flow in order to enhance the effect of radioimmunotherapy. This can be achieved in animal models with flavone acetic acid. This drug causes release of tumour necrosis factor alpha in tumour blood vessels resulting in thrombosis and tumour necrosis. In experimental models this has little effect on tumour growth which rapidly recovers due to reintroduction of blood supply from the tumour periphery. However, in combination with radioimmunotherapy which particularly damages the tumour periphery the therapeutic effect is greatly enhanced. This effect is also produced by methyl xanthenone acetic acid [8]. Clinical trials when radiolabelled antibody and FAA are in progress.

GENETICALLY ENGINEERED ANTIBODIES

Another approach is to genetically engineer antibodies in order to enhance their therapeutic potential. Both reduction in size of the antibody molecule and increase in affinity appear to enhance the tumour to normal tissue ratio and increase penetration through the tumour mass. Clinical studies with a F(ab′)2 antibody (100kD MW) show more rapid penetration tumour by comparison with whole IgG (150kD MW) [7]. A genetically engineered single chain Fv antibody (27kD MW) directed against CEA [9] shows good tumour to normal tissue contrast as soon as 4 h after injection in a clinical imaging study. This antibody was produced from an antibody library expressed in filamentous phage (see separate paper by Dr KA Chester). Antibodies of mouse origin can be humanised by exchanging all but complementarity determining (antigen binding) regions for human antibody components thus reducing their immunogenicity and permitting repeated therapy [10]. Antibody fragments can be linked using synthetic linkers to enhance their stability *in vivo* and increase their valency [10]. These and many other products are being brought towards clinical trials. There are many considerations regarding the quality and safety of antibody produced by protein engineering using recombinant DNA technology and these have been described for application in phase I trials in patients with cancer [11].

CONCLUSION

Antibody targeted therapy can cause tumour responses in patients with colorectal carcinoma using first generation monoclonal antibodies linked to beta-emitting radionuclides. A range of technology is applicable to improve this therapy and it is likely that useful therapy for colorectal cancer will be developed.

REFERENCES

1 Boxer GM, Begent RHJ, Kelly AMB, *et al.* Factors influencing variability of localisation of antibodies to carcinoembryonic antigen (CEA) in patients with colorectal carcinoma—implication for radioimmunotherapy. *Br J Cancer* 1992; **65**: 825–31

2 Begent RHJ, Ledermann JA, Green AJ, *et al.* Antibody distribution and dosimetry in patients receiving radiolabelled antibody therapy for colorectal cancer. *Br J Cancer* 1989; **60**: 406–12

3 Marshall D, Pedley RB, Boden JA, Boden R, Begen RHJ. Clearance of circulating radio-antibodies using streptavidin or second antibody in a xenograft model. *Br J Cancer* 1994; **69**: 502–7

4 Pedley RB, Boden JA, Boden R, Dale R, Begent RHJ. Comparative radioimmunotherapy using intact or F(ab')$_2$ fragments of 131I anti-CEA antibody in a colonic xenograft model. *Br J Cancer* 1993; **68**: 69–73

5 Green AJ, Dewhurst SE, Begent RHJ, Bagshawe KD, Riggs SJ. Accurate quantification of 131I distribution by gamma camera imaging. *Eur J Nucl Med* 1990; **16**: 361–5

6 Leicher PK, Koral KF, Joszcak RJ, Green AJ, Chen GT, Roeske JC. An overview of imaging techniques and physical aspects of treatment planning in radioimmunotherapy. *Med Phys* 1993; **20**: 2

7 Lane DM, Eagle KF, Begent RHJ, *et al. Br J Cancer* 1994; **70**: 521–5

8 Pedley RB, Begent RHJ, Boden JA, Boxer GM, Boden R, Keep PA. Enhancement of radioimmunotherapy by drugs modifying tumour blood flow in a colonic xenograft model. *Int J Cancer* 1994; **57**: 830–5

9 Chester KA, Begent RHJ, Robson L, *et al.* Phage libraries for generation of clinically useful antibodies. *Lancet* 1994; **343**: 455–6

10 King DJ, Mountain A, Adair JR, *et al.* Cancer Research Campaign Operation Manual for Control Recommendations for Product Derived from Recombinant DNA Technology Prepared for Investigational Administration to Patients with Cancer in Phase I Trials. *Eur J Cancer* 1993; **29A**: 1907–10

11 Begent RHJ, Chester KA, Connors T, *et al.* Cancer Research Campaign. Operation manual for control recommendations for product derived from recombinant DNA technology prepared for investigational administration to patients with cancer in Phase I trials. *Eur J Cancer* 1993; **29A**: 1907–10

Considerations in linker design for antibody targeted calicheamicins

Lois M. Hinman and Philip R. Hamann

Lederle Research Division, American Home Products, Pearl River, NY 10965, USA

Over the past several years, we have developed strategies for linking calicheamicins to monoclonal antibodies (MoAbs) and other carrier proteins. Currently, two lead calicheamicin conjugates are under clinical development as the part of the American Cyanamid-Celltech collaborative programme, both incorporating fully humanised MoAbs prepared by CDR-grafting [1]. One conjugate utilises a humanised version of CT-M-01 (hCT-M-01), an antibody which recognises a polymorphic epithelial mucin antigen, abundant on a number of carcinomas of epithelial origin, including breast and ovarian cancers [1]. This conjugate is currently under development for the treatment of ovarian cancer. The second conjugate utilises a humanised version of P67.6 (hP67.6), an anti-CD33 MoAb for treatment of acute myelogenous leukaemia (AML). CD33 is a 67 kD glycoprotein expressed on normal and leukaemic myeloid colony forming cells but not on normal pluripotent haematopoietic stem cells or other normal tissues [3]. Greater than 90% of AML patients express the CD33 antigen on the leukaemic cell population. Clinical studies with iodinated murine P67.6 demonstrate that this MoAb is selective for CD33-positive cells which rapidly and efficiently internalise it after binding [4]. The calicheamicin analogue, N-acetyl gamma 1^I calicheamicin was chosen for linking to both MoAbs. However, based on preclinical data, different linkers appear to be optimal for the two MoAbs. The rationale for the choice of linkers selected for these lead conjugates will be reviewed in this presentation.

N-acetyl gamma 1^I calicheamicin which is used to construct these conjugates is a member of the calicheamicin family of antitumour antibiotics [5]. The calicheamicins were identified based on their impressive potency in a screen for DNA damaging agents, and were later characterised as members of the ene-diyne class of antibiotics which includes the esperamicins, dynemicin, and neocarzinostatin [6]. The binding of the most potent of the calicheamicins, gamma 1^I, in the minor groove of DNA and the resulting sequence-specific DNA cleavage has been reported [7,8]. No members of the calicheamicin family have as yet been developed as stand-alone drugs. Based on the impressive potency of this drug class, however, development of conjugated forms of N-acetyl calicheamicin gamma 1^I is proceeding [9].

Our approach to conjugating the calicheamicins involves converting the methyl trisulphide side chains of the calicheamicins into linker-containing disulphide derivatives, ready for attachment to functional groups on proteins or other macromolecular carriers [10]. As a part of the preclinical development programme, calicheamicin conjugates using murine versions of the lead MoAbs, CT-M-01 and P67.6, with hydrolysable (hydrazone) and non-hydrolysable (amide) type linkages were prepared and compared for selectivity and efficacy *in vitro* and *in vivo*.

We have previously described the potent antitumour effects of carbohydrate-linked conjugates of N-acetyl gamma 1^I calicheamicin-dimethyl-hydrazide with the murine version of CT-M-01 (CT-M-01-N-Ac-DM-Hyd) in models of breast carcinoma [11]. Similarly, amide-linked conjugates prepared with an activated hydroxysuccinimide (OSu) ester of N-acetyl gamma 1^I calicheamicin dimethyl acid (CT-M-01-N-Ac-DM-Amide) have shown comparable activities and specificities to the corresponding hydrazide-linked conjugates in most *in vitro* and *in vivo* models [12]. Both the amide and hydrazone linking technologies produced murine CT-M-01 conjugates with drug loadings of 2.5 to 3.0 molecules of calicheamicin per MoAb, which retained at least 80% the immunoaffinity of the unmodified MoAb. Based on considerations of synthetic ease, yield, potency and stability, the amide linking procedure was applied to the preparation of a humanised CT-M-01 conjugate. This hCT-M-01-N-Ac-DM-Amide conjugate has shown excellent biological activity in preclinical models and is currently in clinical development.

Similarly, hydrazone and amide linked conjugates of murine P67.6 were compared in *in vitro* and *in vivo* models [13]. Unlike CT-M-01 conjugates, conjugates of P67.6 prepared with the hydrolysable hydrazone linkage (P67.6-N-Ac-DM-Hyd) were significantly more active than those prepared with the non-hydrolysable amide linkage (P67-N-Ac-Amide). *In vitro*, the P67.6-N-Ac-DM-Hyd conjugate showed excellent cutotoxicity toward antigen-positive HL-60 cells (mean $IC50=0.20 \pm 0.14$ ng drug equivalents/ml) with 250-fold less potency toward antigen negative Raji cells ($IC50=49.4 \pm 21.9$ ng/ml) ($n=9$). In contrast the IC_{50} for an amide-linked conjugate was >2500 ng/ml toward antigen positive cells under equivalent assay conditions, despite excellent retention of immunoaffinity. *In vivo*, the P67.6-N-Ac-DM-Hyd conjugate inhibited the growth of the HL-60 tumour implanted in nude mice over a six-fold dose range. Under conditions in which the hydrazone conjugate produced 12 tumour-free survivors out of 18 treated animals at 42 days post-treatment, the amide-linked conjugate produced a maximum tumour-inhibition of 80%, with no tumour-free survivors at day 42. P67.6-N-Ac-DM-Hyd was also significantly more active than P67.6-N-Ac-Amide in selectively inhibiting the growth of leukaemic colony cells from patients *ex vivo*. These data suggest that a hydrolysable linker is important for the activity of the P67.6 conjugate in leukaemic cells.

When the carbohydrate-based (hydrazone) linker technology was applied to the humanised version of P67.6, however, significant losses in immunoaffinity were seen due to the antibody's sensitivity to oxidation. As predicted from the murine MoAb data, poor antitumour effects were seen with the amide-linked humanised conjugate, despite excellent retention of immunoaffinity. Based on these results, a programme was undertaken to develop linkers which have the hydrolytic cleavability of the carbohydrate-based hydrazide linker, but do not require an oxidative step in their preparation. A series of new 'hybrid' linkers which contain a hydrolytically cleavable site, but attach to MoAb lysines via amide bonds were prepared, and a lead linker selected for the hP67.6 conjugate. Impressive antitumour activities in preclinical models were seen with this hP67-N-

Ac-DM-Hybrid conjugate, similar to activites seen for the P67.6-N-Ac-DM-Hyd conjugate.

In conclusion, the preclinical studies carried out with two different MoAbs suggest that considerations of linker chemistry are important in designing effective MoAb conjugates with potent cytotoxic agents. Variations in the nature of the target tumour and antibody trafficking patterns that might be predictive of the need for a hydrolysable linker in these conjugates will be discussed.

REFERENCES

1   Hinman LM, Yarranton G. New approaches to non-immunogenic monoclonal antibody cancer therapies. *Ann Rep Med Chem* 1993; **28**: 237–46

2   Aboud-Pirak E, Sergent T, Otte-Slachmuylder C, Abarca J, Trouet A, Schneider Y-J. Binding and endocytosis of a monoclonal antibody to a high molecular weight human milk fat globule membrane-associated antigen by cultured MCF-7 breast cancer cells. *Cancer Res* 1988; **48**: 3188–96

3   Bernstein ID, Singer JW, Andrews RG, *et al.* Treatment of acute myeloid leukemia cells in vitro with a monoclonal antibody recognizing a myeloid differentiation antigen allows normal progenitor cells to be expressed. *J Clin Invest* 1987; **79**: 1153–60

4   Applebaum FR, Matthews DC, Eary JF, *et al.* The use of radiolabeled anti-CD33 antibody to augment marrow irradiation prior to marrow transplantation for acute myelogenous leukemia. *Transplantation* 1992; **54**: 829–33

5   Lee MD, Dunne TM, Chang CC, Morton GO, Borders DB. Calicheamicins, a novel family of antitumor antibiotics, 1: Chemistry and partial characterization of $\gamma 1^I$. *J Am Chem Soc* 1987; **109**: 3464–6

6   Zein N, Ding WD, Ellestad G. Interaction of calicheamicin with DNA. In: Pullman B and Portner J, eds. *Molecular basis of specificity in nucleic acid-drug interactions*, New York: Kluwer Academic Publishers, 1990: 323–30

7   Zein N, Sinha AM, McGahren WJ, Ellestad GA. Calicheamicin $\gamma 1^I$: An antibiotic that cleaves double stranded DNA site specifically. *Science* 1988; **240**: 1198–201

8   Zein N, Poncin M, Nilakantan R, Ellestad G. Calicheamicin $\gamma 1^I$ and DNA: Molecular recognition process responsible for site-specificity. *Science* 1989; **244**: 697–9

9   Lee M, Durr F, Hinman L, Hamann P, Ellestad G. The Calicheamicins In: Maryanoff BE, Maryanoff CA, eds. *Advances in medicinal chemistry*, Greenwich, CT: JAI Press, 1993: 31-66

10 Hinman LM, Hamann PR, Upeslacis J. Preparation of conjugates to monoclonal antibodies. In: Borders D, Doyle T,

eds. *Enediyne antibiotics and antitumor agents*. Marcel Dekker, Inc. 1995; 87–105

11 Hinman LM, Hamann PR, Wallace R, Menendez AT, Durr FE, Upeslacis, J. The preparation and characterization of monoclonal antibody conjugates of the calicheamicins: a novel family of antitumor antibiotics. *Cancer Res* 1993; **53**: 3336–42

12 Hinman LM, Hamann PR, Beyer CF, *et al*. Lysine-linked conjugates of calicheamicins with a fully humanized antipolymorphic epithelial mucin antibody show potent antitumor effects in ovarian tumor xenografts. *Proceedings of the American Association for Cancer Research* 1993; **34**: 479

13 Hinman LM, Hamann PR, Beyer CF, *et al*. Calicheamicin conjugates of the anti-CD33 antibody, P67, show potent, selective antitumor effects in models of acute myeloid leukemia (AML) and against human leukemic bone marrow cells. *Proceedings of the American Association for Cancer Research* 1994; **35**: 507

Immunotoxins in cancer therapy

Peter L. Amlot

Departments of Clinical Immunology and Clinical Oncology, Royal Free Hospital Medical School, London, UK

Many immunotoxins have been used to treat human malignancies, mostly in Phase I studies. The immunotoxins have been constructed from a wide variety of IgG monoclonal antibodies and a range of toxins such as ricin, saporin, pseudomonas exotoxin and pokeweed antiviral protein. The responses to immunotoxin therapy in non-lymphoid tumours have been infrequent and restricted to minor or partial responses. Superior therapeutic results have been obtained treating lymphoid malignancies. The responses are mostly partial but also include a number of complete responses. The clinical responses have generally been short lived.

An important advantage of immunotoxins over radioisotope methods of targeting has been the low level of haematological toxicity seen with their use. There are individual toxicity profiles that differ between the various toxin conjugates. However, all of them cause a dose dependent vascular leak syndrome that appears to be determined by the duration that immunotoxins remain above certain threshold blood concentrations. The other distinctive side effect of immunotoxins is myalgia, mostly of mild intensity but occasionally leading to rhabdomyolysis. Human antibody responses to monoclonal antibodies and to attached toxins occur equally frequently and depend on the degree of the patient's underlying immunosuppression. As long as an immunogenic toxin is attached to the targeting antibody there is little advantage to chimerising or humanising the antibody.

The combination of low haematological toxicity, a unique method of cytotoxicity and inhibition of protein synthesis that may inhibit mechanisms of drug resistance makes immunotoxins particularly appropriate for combination with conventional cytotoxic drugs.

Immunohistochemistry in the characterisation of breast cancer

Rosemary A. Walker

University of Leicester, Breast Cancer Research Unit, Clinical Sciences, Glenfield Hospital, Leicester, UK

Immunohistochemistry has been used increasingly over the past 20 years as a method for analysing the nature of many human tumours and breast cancer is no exception. The introduction of monoclonal antibody technology has extended the range of markers which can be studied and the development of improved detection systems has led to greater applicability.

Immunohistochemistry can provide information of value with regard to treatment and prognosis of breast cancer, but it is important to understand the pros and cons of the technique if it is to be used routinely to provide clinical information.

ADVANTAGES AND DISADVANTAGES OF IMMUNOHISTOCHEMISTRY

Immunohistochemistry can be applied to both cytological specimens and tissue sections. The latter may be either small biopsies or the resected cancer. It can, therefore, be used to gain information of value in selecting therapy to be given either before or instead of surgery. The applicability to small amounts of tissue is an advantage over biochemical techniques. A further advantage is that, in many instances, it can be applied to routinely fixed and processed surgical material whereas biochemical methods for studying proteins require fresh tissue. The number of cancers which can be characterised is therefore much greater.

Immunohistochemical staining of tissue sections gives precise localisation regarding the site of expression. This is particularly important in the screening of monoclonal antibodies which are to be used for treatment purposes, when binding of the antibody should be confined to malignant cells. It is also important when a marker may be within the malignant and the stromal cells in a tumour. A good example of this is cathepsin D which can be present in both of these cell types. Reactivity within them can be distinguished by immunohistochemistry but not by techniques which rely on homogenisation of tissue. Immunohistochemistry also provides information about the heterogeneity of expression within a given cancer.

Once optimised it is a relatively easy technique to perform. Interpretation requires experience but this can be gained.

One of the main disadvantages is that it tends to be qualitative rather than quantitative. It is possible to count the number of cells staining for a particular marker and express this as a percentage. For certain proteins, such as oestrogen receptor, schemes have been devised that incorporate assessment of intensity of staining as well as number of cells reacting. The problems with these are in standardisation of what is 'weak', 'moderate' and 'strong' and in the length of time it takes to do the counting. Image analysis provides a more accurate method but this equipment is expensive, labour intensive and only available in a small number of laboratories.

Immunohistochemistry cannot provide information about the molecular weight or the activity of the antigen which has been detected.

FACTORS IN IMMUNOHISTOCHEMISTRY

The first essential is the availability of specific antibodies. This is less of a problem now since there are many suppliers and monoclonal antibodies overcome the problems of polyclonal antisera.

The next is whether the marker of interest can be detected in routine formalin-fixed tissue. This, again, is less of a problem for several reasons. Antibodies are now developed to react with epitopes in fixed tissue. The methods for revealing antigen sites have increased. Previously these relied on the use of enzymes such as trypsin, pepsin or protease but methods now include the use of microwaves, with sections immersed in citrate buffer, and pressure cookers.

There are various detection systems. Streptavidin-biotin methods provide sensitivity and flexibility.

One of the main factors is standardisation with good quality control, if immunohistochemistry is to be used by many laboratories for clinical applications.

CHARACTERISATION OF BREAST CANCER

The main areas in which immunohistochemistry can be of value are:

- determination of markers which can help in selection of appropriate therapy.
- characterisation of potential behaviour of breast carcinomas. This is of particular value and is associated with selection of therapy if established prognostic factors such as node status are not available.
- assessment of whether tumour-associated antibodies which may be used in serum assays for monitoring recurrence and/or for therapy react with individual breast cancers.

The following section describes a range of receptors, growth factors, oncoproteins, tumour suppressor proteins, proliferation markers plus others which can be detected by immunohistochemistry.

Oestrogen receptor

The original methods for determining oestrogen receptor were biochemical, requiring large amounts of fresh tumour. Antibodies to oestrogen receptor were developed in the 1980s and were important in that the immunohistochemical staining showed the receptor to be nuclear and not cytoplasmic as had been presumed from previous studies. Immunohistochemical analysis also had the advantage of demonstrating heterogeneity of receptor within carcinomas. There was a good correlation between the immunohistochemical and the dextran-coated charcoal techniques and with enzyme immunoassays. The antibodies which were first available required frozen tissue but the use of different enzyme digestion methods made it possible to

detect oestrogen receptor in fixed tissue. The more recently marketed antibodies work well on fixed tissue when used with antigen retrieval methods such as microwaving.

The problems of quantification have already been referred to.

Oestrogen receptor can be detected in fine needle aspirates by immunohistochemistry and is therefore of great value in determining therapy in particular groups of patients.

Progesterone receptor

This is induced by oestrogen and so is a marker of a functioning receptor. The presence of both oestrogen and progesterone receptors is a good guide for the likely response of a cancer to hormone therapy. The original methods for determination were biochemical, similar to oestrogen receptor. The antibodies developed show the receptor to be nuclear. The various antibodies available at work on fixed tissue as frozen and can be applied to cytology specimens.

pS2

The search for other proteins which are induced by oestrogen and could be markers of response to endocrine therapy led to the identification of pS2. This is a small protein, which may be a growth factor. It can be detected immunohistochemically in fixed tissue and cytological specimens. Prominent staining is a useful marker of endocrine responsiveness.

Epidermal growth factor receptor

Overexpression of epidermal growth factor receptor is found in about a third of breast cancers and is inversely related to oestrogen receptor. Cancers are more likely to respond to chemotherapy. Epidermal growth factor receptor can be detected immunohistochemically but the majority of antibodies only work on frozen tissue.

Cathepsin D

The original studies of breast cancer lines indicated that this lysosomal protease was oestrogen regulated. However, in primary carcinomas there is no significant relationship with oestrogen receptor. Analysis of breast cancer homogenates by immunoassay suggested that cathepsin D was a marker of invasion and poor prognosis but immunohistochemical studies have been less conclusive. This may be because the latter method allows localisation and assessment of the different cell types containing cathepsin D (macrophages as well as/instead of cancer cells) whereas all will be included in homogenates.

c-erbB₂

This is also known as neu and HER-2. It is an oncoprotein which is overexpressed in 10–30% of invasive carcinomas. It shows homology with epidermal growth factor receptor. Amplification of the gene and overexpression show a good correlation and the overexpression can be detected in formalin-fixed tissues by immunohistochemistry. In many studies overexpression is an independent marker of poor prognosis.

c-erbB₂ can be detected in about 60% of cases of ductal carcinoma *in situ*, particularly the high grade comedo type but it has not been found in premalignant lesions.

p53

Abnormalities of the p53 gene are important in many cancers. The wild-type protein has a short half life and is not detected by immunohistochemistry but many mutations stabilise the protein so that it can be detected.

p53 illustrates the problems which can occur in interpreting the significance of immunohistochemical staining. DNA damage can lead to increased levels of normal protein and staining. Fixation, tissue processing temperature and detection methods, such as antigen retrieval, can also modify the stability of the protein. Other problems include determining what is the level of significant staining. Despite these problems several studies have shown a relationship between p53 staining and poorer differentiation and poorer prognosis.

Cell proliferation

The proliferation of breast cancers can be a guide for response to therapy and prognosis. There are antibodies to several different components of the cell cycle but in breast the one that provides the most reliable information is Ki-67. This detects cells which are in the cell cycle. It could only be applied to frozen tissue but there are now Ki-67 antibodies which work on fixed tissue with antigen retrieval. Several studies have shown Ki-67 to provide prognostic information.

Angiogenesis

Immunohistochemical determination of microvessel density in the most active areas of neovascularisation of breast cancers have been found to be an independent marker of relapse and survival.

Other markers

The immunohistochemical determination of glycoprotein and enzymes involved in multidrug resistance could be of therapeutic benefit.

The nm23 gene has been identified as a potential metastasis suppressor. Expression of the nm23H1 isotype has been shown to be inversely associated with the presence of nodal metastasis. Care has to be taken about the specificity of antibodies used since no association is found for nm23H2.

CONCLUSIONS

With the recent advancements immunohistochemistry can be used to provide a wealth of information about the nature of breast cancers from quite small samples and from routinely processed tissue. It, therefore, has many advantages, but as with any technique, results are only as good as the care that is taken in performing them and in their interpretation.

Breast cancer antibody imaging

W. J. B. Smellie and Nigel P. M. Sacks*

*Royal Marsden Hospital, Downs Road, Sutton, Surrey,
and *St George's Hospital, Blackshaw Road, London, UK*

INTRODUCTION

Breast cancer is a common disease of women world-wide and is increasing in frequency in the western world [1]. Alongside this increase in frequency of the disease has come an increase in public awareness of the opportunities for early diagnosis and a concomitant increase in expectation of cure. Although the exact benefits of early detection of breast cancer are as yet unclear it nevertheless is generally accepted that the greatest chance in reducing the death rate by early detection of breast cancer will rely on imaging techniques rather than improvements in screening by clinical examination or self-examination, as well as identification of patients at increased risk of breast cancer and cancer prophylaxis [2]. Antibody directed imaging has been used experimentally in the primary detection of breast cancer for a number of years however for a variety of reasons no antibody-imaging technique has yet been developed that is sufficiently accurate to be considered as a candidate to detect early breast cancer or axillary lymph node metastases.

It is not the primary cancer but subsequent metastatic disease that is the cause of mortality and morbidity and it is in the field of detection of these that antibody directed imaging may have a role to play. Although the pattern of spread of breast cancer is notoriously unpredictable, it is usual for the axillary lymph nodes to be involved before systemic spread is detectable or present. Those patients who have involved lymph nodes at the time of presentation have an increased mortality rate from the disease and it is therefore desirable to know the nodal status of all patients to assist in the planning of further management and counselling the patient [3].

Currently the only certain way of assessing the axillary status of patients is to perform axillary staging surgery and this is therefore routinely performed on patients without other evidence of poor prognosis in most breast centres. Axillary dissection may also improve survival as well as giving important prognostic information [4]. The technique is associated with a certain amount of morbidity, as well as an increase in length of hospital stay. As the National Breast Screening Programme continues the number of patients detected with small, clinically impalpable tumours will increase and these early tumours are associated with a low frequency of axillary nodal involvement at presentation. These patients present the surgeon with a dilemma as to whether the morbidity associated with axillary dissection is warranted.

For these reasons there is a definite requirement of reliable non-invasive staging of the axilla. Ultrasound, CT and MRI have all been shown to be able to detect axillary disease however none is accurate enough to be generally accepted as an alternative to axillary dissection. This is therefore a major potential role in the use of antibody-directed imaging and has been fairly extensively investigated at a number of institutions including our own [5–11]. Despite some success with the antibody imaging in cases of breast cancer the technique has not yet been found to be sensitive enough to be routinely used. There are a variety of reasons for this, many of which are common to all antibody detected therapy and a few specially so in the case of breast cancer.

TARGET ANTIGENS

Perhaps the most frustrating aspect of antibody directed imaging and therapy of breast cancer is the absence of a specific, universally expressed antigen on the cell surface of all breast cancers. Most breast cancer cells, in common with other epithelial cell carcinomas, express common epithelial membrane antigen (EMA) and this, along with human milk fat globulin has been the most favoured target in human trials of imaging of breast cancers [5,8–19]. Neither is specific to breast cancer cells and therefore the quality of images using antibodies directed against these antigens is bound to be poor. Alternative much more specific antigens that are over-expressed in around 30% of breast cancer are c-erbB$_2$p185 and the epidermal growth factor receptor (EGFR) and these have been the target for our imaging [6]. Both are growth factor receptors in the tyrosine kinase group and are structurally partially homologous. C-erbB$_2$ antigen expression is associated with poor response to chemotherapy [20], endocrine therapy [21] and poor overall prognosis [22,23]. It is therefore highly suitable as a target for antibody directed imaging and therapy studies, since an increased number of patients who express this antigen will have involved axillary nodes and disseminated disease. The antigen has been well characterised and several monoclonal antibodies are now available of clinical grade for use in patient trials [24]. These antibodies are of varying specificity recognising different epitopes on the external domain of the antigen, both the protein core which is highly specific to the antigen and minimally expressed in normal adult tissues and also against glycoprotein associated with the antigen. Antibodies directed against these parts of the antigen are less specific and may cross-react with carbohydrate moieties in other sites such as the lung and are therefore less suitable for human trials, since the whole value of using anti-cerbB$_2$ antibodies rather than common antigens such as EMA is their specificity.

ICR12 is a rat-derived IgG$_{2a}$ monoclonal antibody against the external domain of the c-erbB$_2$p185 protein core. It has a high Ka binding (0.2nM) and is highly specific to breast cancer cells in patients who overexpress the antigen. For this reason we have been using this antibody in clinical trials of imaging of breast cancer [6]. Only 20–30% of breast cancers overexpress the antigen which represents a major draw-back in the use of this antibody however fortunately it is possible to predict in advance of imaging any patient whether their tumours are of the subclass that overexpress c-erbB$_2$ by immunohistochemical staining of the fine-needle aspirate cytology specimens or core-cut biopsies that are routinely obtained prior to surgery as a fundamental diagnostic procedure in any patient with a palpable breast lump (25). Finally in patients undergoing needle-guided biopsy of screen detected lesions who are found to have c-erbB$_2$ overexpressing tumours, post-operative axillary imaging may identify the occasional

unexpected axillary regional spread that would not be recognised since these patients often do not have axillary surgery as a staged procedure and therefore identify those screen-detected patients with breast cancer who might benefit from adjuvant chemotherapy. We believe therefore that the benefits of using antibodies against c-erbB$_2$ for studies of imaging in patients with breast cancer outweigh the disadvantage of the lack of universal expression of the antigen. Success with the use of this antibody in the radio imaging and radioimmunotherapy of breast cancer should be an added incentive to search for a universally expressed, specific breast cancer antigen.

ROUTE OF ADMINISTRATION

A variety of routes of administration of radiolabelled antibodies are available, of which intravenous is the most attractive because of its simplicity. Unfortunately with breast cancers, as with almost all other solid tumours, the blood flow to deposits is relatively poor and may be a critical factor in the success of the technique. This may be particularly true of axillary nodal deposits which are suspended in the adipose tissue of the axilla and are often found at surgery to be necrotic due to outgrowth of the vascular supply. An alternative used for radioimmunotherapy has been the direct intralesional injection of the radiopharmaceutical agent however this route is obviously not possible in the primary radioimmunodetection of lesions. The propensity of breast cancer to deposit primarily in axillary lymph nodes prior to systemic dissemination has the advantage that the intralymphatic route can be utilised and indeed this route has been successfully used in a number of reported studies [5,8,26] although false positives are a problem.

ISOTOPES AND IMAGING MODALITIES

The majority of human imaging trials have used either ^{99m}Tc or ^{111}In as the isotopes because of their easy availability and suitability for planar or SPECT imaging and relatively short half-lives allowing large radiation doses to be given. Positron emission tomogram (PET) imaging allows quantifiable imaging of monoclonal antibodies in tumour deposits with a resolution of 0.5–1 cm, reducing the size of tumours that can be visualised [27,28]. Positron emitting isotopes must be used, which are only recently becoming widely available. We have studied patients with breast cancer using ^{124}I labelled ICR12 and have been impressed by the quality of the images obtained. A further advantage of using this isotope is that the chemistry of conjugation and excretion of this imaging isotope is the same as for a potential therapeutic isotope ^{131}I. It remains to be seen whether this technique is able to detect deposits with sufficient sensitivity and specificity to be useful in the diagnosis and staging of the axilla in patients with breast cancer however the initial results suggest that it will not.

IMAGING STUDIES AS TOOLS FOR DOSIMETRY IN INDIVIDUAL PATIENTS

The most interesting application in the field of radio-immunodetection is dosimetry prior to radioimmunotherapy. Early results of this form of therapy were disappointing largely because some patients failed to localise the radiopharmaceutical despite having tumours that expressed the antigen target. A variety of reasons for this failure to localise have been proposed, including the poor blood supply of a particular deposit and raised intra-tumour interstitial pressure. For this reason a number of patients have received therapeutic doses of isotopes that did not have any effect on the primary tumour however risked myelotoxicity. Imaging the tumours prior to administration of the radioisotope is a favoured method of confirming the ability of the conjugate to localise and is a valuable adjunct to the MIRD tables in predicting the actual tumour uptake and dose of ionising radiation [29]. The PET scanner can give accurate uptake dose estimates of the amount of activity of a test dose of positron emitting isotope, which is able to estimate the %ID/l within the tumour and also the dose to non-tumour organs to estimate side-effects of therapy. In our most recent patient scanned using ICR12 and ^{124}I label we calculated, using 1st order MIRD estimates, that with a single dose of 600MBq of ^{131}I intravenously we might expect 36Gy to the tumour without excess marrow toxicity. Further information will come available from this technique that will allow us to assess whether labelled ICR12 may be useful in the treatment of metastatic breast cancer.

REFERENCES

1 Harris JR, Lippman ME, Veronesi U, Willett W. Breast cancer. *N Engl J Med* 1993; **327**: 319–28, 390–98, 473–80

2 Powles TJ, Tillyer CR, Jones A, *et al.* Prevention of breast cancer with tamoxifen—an update of the Royal Marsden Hospital pilot programme. *Eur J Cancer* 1990; **26**: 680–4

3 Sacks NPM, Barr LC, Allan SM, Baum M. The role of axillary dissection in operable breast cancer. *The Breast* 1992; **1**: 41–9

4 Axelsson CK, Mouridsen HT, Zedeler K. Axillary dissection of level 1 and 11 lymph nodes is important in breast cancer classification. *Eur J Cancer* 1992; **28A**: 1415–18

5 Tjandra JJ, Sacks NPM, Thompson CH, *et al.* The detection of axillary lymph node metastases from breast cancer by radiolabelled monoclonal antibodies: a prospective study. *Br J Cancer* 1989; **59**: 296–302

6 Allan SM, Dean C, Fernando I, *et al.* Radioimmunolocalisation in breast cancer using the gene product of c-erbb2 as the target antigen. *Br J Cancer* 1993; **67**: 706–12

7 Dean CJ, Allan SM, Eccles S, *et al.* The product of the c-erbB2 proto-oncogene as a target for diagnosis and therapy in breast cancer. In: Cruse JM, Lewis RE, eds. *The year in immunology*. 7th ed. Basel, Switzerland: S. Karger, 1993: 182–92

8 Tjandra JJ, Russell IS, Collins JP, *et al.* Immunolymphoscintigraphy for the detection of lymph node metastases from breast cancer. *Cancer Res* 1989; **49**: 1600–8.

9 Couto JR, Blank EW, Peterson JA, Ceriani RL. Cloning of cDNAs encoding the variable domains of antibody BrE-3 and construction of a chimeric antibody. *Hybridoma* 1993; **12**: 15–23

10 Pecking AP, Bertrand FJ, Lokiec FM, *et al.* Preoperative immunolymphoscintigraphy with human monoclonal antibody (16-88 LiLo) to assess the nodal involvement in breast cancer (Meeting abstract). *Fourth Annual Symposium: Current Status and Future Directions of Immunoconjugates.* 1992

11 Lamki LM, Buzdar AU, Singletary SE, *et al.* Indium-111-labeled B72.3 monoclonal antibody in the detection and staging of breast cancer: A phase I study. *J Nucl Med* 1991; **32**: 1326–32

12 Biersack HJ, Hotze AL, Schultes B, Bender H, Schomburg A, Grunwald F. Clinical relevance of radio-immunoimaging in malignant diseases. *Onkologie* 1993; **16**: 222–9

13 Kramer EL, DeNardo SJ, Liebes L, *et al.* Radioimmunolocalization of metastatic breast carcinoma using indium-111- methyl benzyl DTPA BrE-3 monoclonal antibody: Phase I study. *J Nucl Med* 1993; **34**: 1067–74

14 Reske S, Kartsens J, Sohn M, Glockner W, Buell U. Bone marrow immunoscintigraphy compared with conventional bone scintigraphy for the detection of bone metastases. *Acta Oncol* 1993; **32**: 753–61

15 Kramer EL. Radioimmunodetection of breast cancer (Meeting abstract). *Fourth Annual Symposium: Current Status and Future Directions of Immunoconjugates.* 1992; -3, 1992

16 DeNardo SJ, O'Grady LF, Macey DJ, *et al.* Quantitative imaging of mouse L-6 monoclonal antibody in breast cancer patients to develop a therapeutic strategy. *Nucl Med Biol Int J Radiat Appl Instrum Part B* 1991; **18**: 621–31

17 Duda RB, Zimmer AM, Rosen ST, *et al.* Radioimmune localization of occult carcinoma. *Arch Surg* 1990; **125**: 866–70

18 Major PP, Dion AS, Williams CJ, Mattes MJ, Wang T, Rosenthall L. Breast tumor radioimmunodetection with a (111)In-labeled monoclonal antibody (MA5) against a mucin-like antigen. *Cancer Res* 1990; **50**: 927–931s

19 Baum RP, Hertel A, Lorenz M, Schwarz A, Encke A, Hor G. (99)Tc(m)-labelled anti-CEA monoclonal antibody for tumour immunoscintigraphy: First clinical results. *Nucl Med Commun* 1989; **10**: 345–52

20 Gusterson BA, Gelber RD, Goldhirsch A, *et al.* Prognostic importance of c-erbB2 expression in breast cancer. *J Clin Oncol* 1992; **10**: 1049–56

21 Wright C, Nicholson S, Angus B, *et al.* Relationship between c-erbB₂ protein product expression and response to endocrine therapy in advanced breast cancer. *Br J Cancer* 1992; **65**: 118–21

22 Anbazhagan R, Gelber RD, Bettelheim R, Goldhirsch A, Gusterson BA. Association of c-erbB₂ expression and s-phase fraction in the prognosis of node positive breast cancer. *Ann Oncol* 1991; **2**: 47–53

23 Gullick WJ, Love SB, Wright C, *et al.* C-erbB₂ protein overexpression in breast cancer is a risk factor in patients with involved and uninvolved lymph nodes. *Br J Cancer* 1991; **63**: 434–8

24 Flower MA, Al Saadi A, McCready VR, *et al.* Dose-response study on thyrotoxic patients undergoing PET and radioiodine therapy (meeting abstract). *Br J Radiol* 1990; **63**: 25

25 Fernando IN, Allan SM, Sandle J, Sacks NPM, Trott PA. The role of fine needle aspirate cytology and the cytospin technique in determination of immunocytochemical staining for the c-erbB₂ gene product. *Cytopath* 1992;

26 Tjandra JJ, Russell IS, Collins JP. Immunolyphoscintigraphy for detection of lymph node metastases from breast cancer. *Cancer Res* 1989; **49**: 1600–8

27 Wilson CB, Snook DE, Dhokia B, *et al.* Quantitative measurement of monoclonal antibody distribution and blood flow using positron emmission tomography and 124Iodine in patients with breast cancer. *Int J Cancer* 1991; **47**: 344–7

28 Ott RJ. The applications of positron emission tomography to oncology [editorial]. *Br J Cancer* 1991; **63**: 5

29 Watson EE, Stabin MG, Siegel JA. MIRD formulation. *Med Phys* 1993; **20**: 511–14

Radioimmunoguided surgery for colorectal cancer

N. A. Theodorou

Charing Cross Hospital, Fulham Palace Road, London, UK

INTRODUCTION

In radioimmunoguided surgery (RIGS™), monoclonal antibodies raised against antigens from colorectal tumours are labelled with ^{125}I and administered to patients after blocking of their thyroid gland to prevent the inappropriate uptake of activity. Patients are submitted to surgery 4–16 days after injection. At operation, the distribution of radioactivity is determined using a 1 cm cadmium telluride hand-held gamma detecting probe (Neoprobe™) with counts being taken in triplicate in particular over the primary tumour, lymphatic field and suspicious areas prior to resection. Following standard radical resections the tumour bed is again scanned for evidence of residual tumour. Finally, the residual specimen is scanned and the counts obtained correlated with the representative samples of tissue, counted in a well counter.

The technique is dependent on the uptake of antibody by the tumour in preference to normal tissue. Hence the selection of antibody to be used is critical. Previous studies have been limited by the limited uptake of antibody by up to only 75% of tumours [1].

THE STUDY

We have looked at three monoclonal antibodies: FM1D10, an antibody to foetal colonic microvillus membrane which has been shown to localise well to human colonic xenographs in nude mice [2]; A5B7, a mouse monoclonal antibody to carcinoembryonic antigen [3] which has been used for external imaging of occult colorectal tumour recurrence; and F(ab′)2, a fragment of A5B7 which it has been suggested shows improved specific localisation.

The aims have been:

1. To determine the best antibody for use in RIGS™

2. To determine the contribution RIGS™ makes to surgical decision making

3. To assess its limitations.

PATIENTS AND TUMOURS

Ninety-one tumours in 83 patients with primary colorectal cancer and nine patients undergoing surgery for recurrent colorectal cancer were studied.

RESULTS

Primary colorectal tumours

The primary tumour

Radioactive counts were taken over the primary tumour and then normal colon, and the results expressed as a ratio of tumour to normal colon counts. In accordance with other studies, ratios of >1.5–1 were taken to be indicative of tumour. A comparison of A5B7, its F(ab′)2 fragment and FM1D10 showed that the best tumour: normal colon ratios were obtained with the fragment (5.6:1) and A5B7 (2.9:1) rather than FM1D10 (1.5:1). The individual tumour: normal colon ratios demonstrated that statistically significant higher ratios were obtained with the fragment when compared to the whole antibody; and the whole antibody when compared to FM1D10 (p<0.001 MWU test). Overall, using A5B7 or its F(ab′)2 fragment between 95–100% of primary tumours localised significant quantities of radioactivity with the ratios >1.5–1, and 80–92% localising with ratios of >2:1. Two out of three patients who did not localise in this group represented technical errors of injection. Only 50% of tumours localised FM1D10 with ratios >1.5:1 and its use was subsequently abandoned.

When the scans were repeated on the resected specimens, the ratios, as might be expected with closer proximity of the probe, revealed even higher ratios (A5B7 5.5:1, F(ab')2 11.8:1, FM1D10 1.9:1) with well counting of representative samples also confirming the significant uptake of radioactivity detected per-operatively by the probe.

The clearance of A5B7 and its F(ab')2 fragment from the blood stream were shown to be virtually identical. It is likely that the superior ratios obtained with the fragment reflected the greater interval between injection and surgery which was adopted when the fragment became available.

Regional lymph nodes

The probe count over the root of the mesentery representing the lymph nodes relating to the primary tumour were compared with the final Dukes' staging. Overall Dukes' C stage was correctly predicted in 14 cases (of 67 that were able to be evaluated) and Dukes' A or B correctly identified in 24 (true negative). There were four false positive readings and 25 false negatives. The overall sensitivity for predicting Dukes' stage was 36%, specificity 85.7% and overall accuracy 57%.

Ex-vivo study of lymph nodes

Seventy-two lymph nodes were individually examined *ex-vivo* with the probe and subjected to detailed histological examination. Tumour metastases were correctly identified by A5B7 in 21/30 nodes. F(ab')2 correctly identified tumour in 40/43 nodes examined. No data were available for FM1D10. The overall sensitivity for predicting nodal histology for A5B7 and F(ab')2 was 72%, specificity 95% and accuracy 86%. There was no significant difference between intact antibody and the fragment for predicting nodal histology (Chi-square=0.913).

Additional clinical information

The RIGS™ system gave additional correct clinical information as confirmed by histological analysis in 20/75 (26.6%) patients. Consequently the management of 6 patients was altered (8%). In nine patients the probe gave incorrect information (12%), but in only one of these was management influenced.

Recurrent colorectal cancer

Nine patients with either local recurrence of colorectal cancer ($n=7$) or metachronous tumours ($n=2$) were also studied using A5B7. This antibody was taken up by the recurrent tumour in ratios >1.5:1 in 8/9 (88%) patients. Additional information was obtained in five patients (55%) and influenced management in three patients (33%). One false negative result was obtained where A5B7 was not taken up by recurrent liver metastases.

CONCLUSIONS

- The monoclonal antibody A5B7 and its F(ab')2 fragment are significantly superior to antibodies previously used in RIGS™, localising significantly in 98.7% of primary tumours and 88% of recurrent cancers.

- Further information was obtained in 26% of patients undergoing primary resections and 53% of patients undergoing second look procedures influencing management in 8% and 33% respectively.

- The accurate identification of lymph node metastases and detection of subclinical diseases requires further evaluation.

REFERENCES

1 O'Dwyer PJ, Sickle-Santarello B, Mojeisik CM, Thurston MD, Martin EW. Intraoperative radioimmunodetection of gastrointestinal neoplasms. *Br J Surg* 1987; **74**: 1145

2 Hennigan T, Carpenter R, Mathews J, *et al*. Regional perfusion of isotope conjugate can increase tumour uptake. *Br J Cancer* 1988; **50**: 530

3 Pedley RB, Boden J, Keep PA, Harwood PJ, Green AJ, Rogers GT. Relationship between tumour size and uptake of radiolabelled anti-CEA in a colon tumour xenograph. *Eur J Nucl Med* 1987; **13**: 197

Vaccines based on tumour antigens

J. Taylor-Papadimitriou
and J. M. Burchell
Imperial Cancer Research Fund, Epithelial Cell Biology Laboratory, London, UK

INTRODUCTION

It is 100 years since William Coley first reported that tumours could be induced to regress under the influence of the immune system activated by bacterial toxins. Although some tantalising data have emerged since then from animal models, there has been little progress in applying immunotherapy to the management of cancer patients. However, the last few years have seen a renewal of interest in the idea of recruiting the defences of the host to reject tumours and clinical trials are now beginning. There are two main reasons for the recent optimism. Firstly, specific tumour-associated antigens have been identified and in many cases, the genes coding for these antigens have been cloned, and secondly much more is known about the molecular mechanisms underlying antigen presentation and the humoral and cellular immune responses. Clearly antigen presentation is of the utmost importance since tumours expressing novel antigens are not rejected, and successful recruitment of the immune system will require improved recognition of the antigen, particularly by T-cells.

ANTIGEN PRESENTATION

Although it is not entirely clear which compartments of the immune system are functional in tumour rejection, cytotoxic T-cells (CTLs) are thought to play a major role in the recognition of tumour antigens and in killing the cells expressing these antigens. It is now known that internal antigens can be presented as peptides by surface HLA-class I molecules to the T-cell receptor. This means that oncogenes involved in intracellular signalling pathways as well as nuclear proteins can all potentially be presented to

the T-cell. Thus the products of mutated genes could be recognised, providing that the presented peptide contains the mutated sequence. Moreover there is evidence to suggest that even normal self antigens can also be recognised, when they are overexpressed.

Much of the work in mouse models, and most of the clinical trials looking to evaluate active specific immunotherapy has been done with melanomas. One reason for this is that they appear to be able to express HLA class II molecules and peptides presented by these class II molecules could activate helper T-cells which then produce cytokines. These cytokines allow the proliferation of the cytotoxic T-cells which have recognised other peptides presented by HLA class I molecules on the tumour cell. The cells in epithelial cancers, i.e. carcinomas are particularly inefficient in antigen presentation, do not express HLA-class II molecules and can lose expression of class I quite frequently. However studies with professional antigen presenting cells (APCs) have led to the identification of molecules, expressed by these cells, which 'co-stimulate' T-cells whose receptor has bound to the peptide-HLA complex on the APC. Thus, the interaction of one of the B7 family of molecules with the CD28 receptor of T-cells has been found to be a necessary co-stimulus for the interaction of the APC with the T-cell receptor to induce IL-2 production and proliferation. If the B7/CD28 interaction occurs along with the engagement of the T-cell receptor then even the cytotoxic T-cell secretes IL-2: without co-stimulus anergy is induced. A corollary of this is that if the B7 molecule is introduced into and expressed by tumour cells (even epithelial tumour cells) their immunogenicity is dramatically enhanced resulting in tumour rejection.

To solve the problem of poor antigen presentation by the carcinoma cell, two alternative strategies may be applied.

53

Where the tumour antigen is well characterised and a cDNA available, ways can be sought to express the antigen in professional APCs. Alternatively, or preferably in addition, cytokines, or co-stimulatory molecules such as B7 may be introduced into the tumour cells. This would result in improved antigen presentation providing HLA class I molecules are being expressed.

IN VITRO AND *IN VIVO* APPROACHES

The above strategies are being applied in various ways both in animal models and in patients. Much of the work involves introducing genes coding for cytokines or B7 into tumour cells *in vitro* and re-introducing these cells into the host, although direct injection of the genes into accessible tumours is also being attempted. Where metastatic sites are not accessible, it may be possible to direct expression of the gene by injecting a DNA based vehicle expressing the cytokine or the co-stimulatory molecule from a specific promoter that restricts expression of the gene to the tumour cells.

Similarly a tumour-specific or tumour-associated antigen may be expressed in APCs cultured *in vitro* using a recombinant retrovirus to obtain efficient expression, and then re-introduced. Although cumbersome as a therapeutic regime, such experiments will give some idea as to whether it is possible to obtain a strong immune response to a particular antigen. Direct injection of the gene coding for a particular antigen or some form of the antigen itself is in the long run a more feasible therapeutic approach and to evaluate the best immunogen for such a protocol animal models are required.

THE POLYMORPHIC EPITHELIAL MUCIN (PEM)

Several tumour associated antigens are under study, including CEA, the MAGE antigens identified by Boon and colleagues on melanoma cells, and oncogenes. We have focused on PEM, the product of the MUC1 gene, which is expressed by more than 90% of breast and ovarian cancers and by a high proportion of other carcinomas, such as lung and colon. PEM is a membrane glycoprotein which is highly glycosylated and normally expressed on the luminal surface of most glandular epithelia. The extracellular domain is made up largely of tandem repeats of 20 amino acids (20–100 depending on the allele) each of which contains potential O-glycosylation sites. In the cancer associated mucin, the core protein is aberrantly glycosylated and as a result the molecule is antigenically distinct from the normal mucin: Novel carbohydrate epitopes appear, and epitopes between glycosylation sites which are normally masked become exposed. Both humoral and cellular responses to PEM have been observed in breast, ovarian and colon cancer patients. The striking feature of the CTLs which have been isolated is that the killing of the target cell is not HLA restricted, and in fact does not require the HLA molecule. The likely explanation for this unusual form of response is that multiple interactions occur between identical epitopes on the extracellular domain of PEM with several T-cell receptors, allowing cross linking and signalling to occur. The molecule is very elongated, and extends way beyond the glycoalyx, and could easily extend around the T-cell. Most of the data with CTLs has come from the laboratory of Oliviera Finn. These studies indicate that the epitope recognised by the T-cell is similar to a core protein epitope (PDTRP) recognised by the antibody SM3 which preferentially reacts with the cancer associated mucin. This suggest that the aberrant glycosylation of PEM results in the antigen—as a membrane glycoprotein—being recognised as non-self.

The lack of requirement for HLA makes PEM an extremely interesting target antigen. Even if the HLA class I molecules are not lost from a cancer cell, a specific peptide will only be presented by a particular allele, making design of vaccine formulations more complex. There are however many possible immunogens based on PEM, which could be used in a vaccine or in active specific immunotherapy. To evaluate the efficacy of the different immunogens and to optimise antigen presentation, animal models are required.

MOUSE MODELS FOR EVALUATION
OF PEM BASED IMMUNOGENS

We have developed both syngeneic and transgenic models for evaluation of MUC1 or PEM based immunogens. In the syngeneic model MUC1 gene has been transfected into mouse tumour cell lines which are transplantable in H2d and H2b mice. These are useful for comparing immunogens for efficacy, for evaluating adjuvants and to test the possibility of using a DNA based vaccine. Several forms of immunogen have been shown to be effective vaccines in this system and specific CTLs have also been observed in immunised mice. The models are limited however because the human MUC1 is a foreign antigen showing only 30% homology with the mouse homologue. The MUC1 transgenic (TG) mouse on the other hand expresses the human gene in the same tissues as it is normally expressed in patients and therefore will show the same tolerance seen in humans. Any autoimmune responses which might occur would also be seen in these animals. The TG mice are therefore appropriate for preclinical toxicity testing. Spontaneous MUC1-expressing tumours have been developed in these mice by cross fostering on an MMTV producing mouse strain and transplantable tumour cell lines are also available for testing different immunogens.

CLINICAL TRIALS WITH PEM BASED ANTIGENS

We have chosen to investigate possible protocols in the mouse models in order to design clinical trials which might have a chance of success. However two trials are ongoing using antigens based on PEM. The first, supported by BIOMIRA is being carried out in various centres, including the ICRF unit at Guy's and uses one of the shorter carbohydrate side chains which may be carried on the cancer-associated mucin.

The second is being carried out in Pittsburgh and uses a polypeptide which covers five tandem repeats of the core protein of PEM. Clearly these phase I trials using patients with established metastic disease are not expected to show dramatic effects on disease progression. They will however give further data on the immune responses which are induced by these particular antigens. It is hoped that in the future, based on the information obtained from both the mouse models and the patient trials, that a PEM based immunogen can be tested in an adjuvant setting where the tumour load is low, preferably together with a strategy where the antigen is presented effectively by both APCs and the cancer cells.

Plasmid vaccination for immunotherapy of lymphoma

Robert E. Hawkins

Centre for Protein Engineering and Department of Clinical Oncology, Addenbrooke's Hospital, Hills Road, Cambridge, UK

Vaccination against malignant disease has long been an attractive prospect but, in contrast to the prevention and treatment of infectious diseases, progress has been slow. The problems encountered include the identification of true tumour-specific targets and the design of suitable vaccines and adjuvants to overcome the (relative) tolerance to tumour antigens. Even if an immune response can be generated there may be problems. For example, T-cells may fail to recognise the tumour antigens because of loss of MHC expression and other defects of antigen processing/presentation in tumour cells. There are less difficulties with humoral immunity if surface targets exist. Various forms of immunotherapy have been tested in a number of malignant diseases but successes have been largely confined to a limited number of diseases including melanoma, renal cell cancer and lymphoma.

A number of features make B-cell lymphoma a particularly attractive prospect for immunotherapy. First, this is the most common type of tumour in immunosuppressed people; second, a true tumour-specific antigen is present on its surface (the idiotypic immunoglobulin) [1]; third, the tumour cells express MHC class 1 and fourth they can be good antigen presenting cells [2]. Furthermore, successes have been achieved with a variety of immunotherapeutic approaches including anti-idiotype monoclonal antibodies [3] and interferon therapy. Although there are many other therapies for malignant lymphoma disseminated low grade tumours are very rarely (if ever) cured and there is little evidence that current treatment prolongs survival. Chemotherapy and radiotherapy produce good symptomatic remissions but with repeated treatment resistant disease emerges and remissions become shorter. There is thus a clear need for new therapies. Since the disease strikes most commonly in the sixth or seventh decade and has a median survival of 8–10 years treatment which has low toxicity seems most appropriate.

The idiotypic immunoglobulin is a specific target for immunotherapy of B-cell lymphoma and extensive trials of anti-idiotype monoclonal antibody therapy have been carried out with overall response rates of 68% [4]. Interestingly this may result from immunologically mediated responses or as a direct result of cross-linking immunoglobulins leading to apoptosis [4]. Tumour escape, however, is possible through somatic mutation and this has been molecularly defined [5]—importantly immunoglobulin loss mutants have not been described. Active immunotherapy through idiotypic vaccination has the attraction over monoclonal antibody therapy that escape from a polyclonal B- and T-cell response will be harder and that persisting immunity may be able to control residual dormant tumour should it subsequently become active. Pioneering work by Levy in Stanford to test this approach has shown that in advanced disease vaccination was unsuccessful but in earlier stage disease the approach is promising with immunological responses and tumour regressions being obtained [6]. This trial utilised conventional cell immortalisation techniques which are unreliable and very time-consuming, bearing in mind that the treatment has to be individualised for each patient. We have been investigating new methods of isolating the tumour derived idiotype and of making such individualised vaccines to facilitate wide application of this approach.

The development of the polymerase chain reaction (PCR) allows the rapid isolation of antibody genes from any source [7]. We use a set of 24 primers to amplify the genes from tumour biopsies. The amplification is followed by cloning and direct sequencing of the products. From normal lymphoid tissue only a random selection of V-genes is obtained but as expected tumour derived tissues contain multiply repeated copies of the tumour associated sequences. Using this process we have been able to isolate tumour derived V_H and V_L from 11/13 B-cell malignancies [8]—in principle this takes less than one week per patient. The failures are probably as a result of poor primer homology and as more information about V-gene sequences emerges it will be possible to design improved primers. The sequencing of V-genes may also give rise to new ways of classifying tumours and of following their clonal development [9].

The most obvious method of generating a vaccine would be to make recombinant protein and use standard immunological adjuvants. We investigated the possibility of using this approach but found that murine scFv's expressed from bacteria were poorly immunogenic in mice. As an alternative we investigated plasmid vaccination. Direct inoculation of plasmid into muscles gives rise to surprisingly high levels of cell transfection and expression can persist for many months [10]. Using this approach as a means of vaccination potentially bypasses the need for recombinant protein production. Initially, a vector which expressed the scFv in fusion with the retroviral envelope protein [11] was used and shown to produce good immunological responses to a murine scFv in mice [12]. These responses could be boosted with recombinant protein or further plasmid vaccination, were specific and the resulting antibody also recognises the native immunoglobulin from which the scFv's were derived [12]. Potentially this approach has additional advantages. As the antigen should also be presented on MHC-class 1 molecules it may be a good method of generating cytotoxic T-cell responses. This has been demonstrated for several foreign proteins [13] but has yet to be demonstrated for a tumour antigen in a syngeneic host.

The initial vectors [11,12] we used were not ideal for patient use as they contained a large component of murine retroviral sequences with the attendant risks of recombination with endogenous retroviruses. For clinical trials new vectors avoiding these problems have been made and tested in mice. The production of plasmid DNA is straightforward and can readily be applied to the production of patient specific products—a feature which would be much harder for recombinant protein approaches. DNA is produced by adaptations of standard

Table 1. Tumour targets for plasmid immunisation

Disease	Target antigen
Cell surface targets	
B-cell malignancies	Immunoglobulin
T-cell malignancies	T-cell receptor
Squamous cell lung cancer	Mutated EGFR
Malignant glioma	Mutated EGFR
Gastric cancer	TPR-MET fusion
Intracellular targets	
Cervical carcinoma	Papilloma virus E6/E7
Many malignancies	Mutant p53/Ras
Melanoma	MAGE/mutated MAGE
?Differentiation antigens	
Colo-rectal cancer	CEA/Muc1
Breast cancer	HER2/Muc1
Squamous cell carcinoma	EGFR
Ovarian carcinoma	CA125

laboratory techniques and can readily be prepared free of protein and endotoxin contamination. A phase I clinical trial is now under way.

The plasmid vaccination approach also allows simple extension by the inclusion of adjuvant molecules to enhance the immune response. It remains to be seen if this will be necessary in the patient situation but certainly patients with advanced disease are somewhat immunosuppressed. The possibilities include the coexpression of cytokines (e.g. IL-2 or GM-CSF) or costimulatory molecules (e.g. B7-1 or B7-2). There is already some indication that they may be of value—IL-2 resulted in an enhanced response to a human immunoglobulin in mice but it also lead to enhanced local tissue destruction [14]. Should other antigens be discovered in B-cell malignancies they could also be simply incorporated into the vaccine design and would reduce the risk of tumour escape though antigenic modulation.

This approach could obviously be applied to other tumours where tumour specific antigens exist. Additionally it may be applicable to the large number of tumour associated antigens identified. However, in such situations the ability of this approach to break tolerance and the possible consequences of this are not known. This will need to be investigated in murine models before patient trials could be contemplated. However, a selection of the possible targets are shown in Table 1.

Acknowledgment

Dr Robert Hawkins is a Cancer Research Campaign senior clinical research Fellow.

REFERENCES

1 Stevenson GT, Stevenson FK. Antibody to molecularly-defined antigen confined to a tumour cell surface. *Nature* 1975; **254**: 714–16

2 Stevenson FK, Hawkins RE. Molecular vaccines against cancer. *The Immunologist* 1994; **2**: 16–19

3 Miller RA, Maloney DG, Warnke R, Levy R. Treatment of B-cell lymphoma with monoclonal anti-idiotype antibody. *N Engl J Med* 1982; **306**: 517–22

4 Vuist WMJ, Levy R, Maloney DG. Lymphoma regression induced by monoclonal anti-idiotypic antibodies correlates with their ability to induce Ig signal transduction and is not prevented by tumour expression of high levels of Bcl-2 protein. *Blood* 1994; **83**: 899–906

5 Bahler DW, Levy R. Clonal evolution of a follicular lymphoma: evidence for antigen selection. *Proc Natl Acad Sci USA* 1992; **89**: 6770–4

6 Kwak LW, Campbell MJ, Czerwinski DK, Hart S, Miller RA, Levy R. Induction of immune responses in patients with B-cell lymphoma against the surface-immunoglobulin idiotype expressed by their tumours. *N Engl J Med* 1992; **327**: 1209–15

7 Ward ES, Güssow D, Griffiths AD, Jones PT, Winter G. Binding activities of a repertoire of single immunoglobulin variable domains secreted from *Escherichia coli*. *Nature* 1989; **344**: 544–6

8 Hawkins RE, Zhu D, Ovecka M, Winter G, Hamblin TJ, Stevenson FK. Idiotypic vaccination against B-cell lymphoma: rescue of variable region gene sequences from biopsy material for assembly as single chain Fv "personal" vaccines. *Blood* 1994; **83**: 3279–88

9 Zhu D, Hawkins RE, Hamblin TJ, Stevenson FK. Clonal history of a human follicular lymphoma as revealed in the immunoglobulin variable region genes. *Br J Haematol* 1994: **86**: 505–12

10 Wolff JA, Malone RW, Williams P, Chong W, Ascadi G, Jani A, Felgner PL. Direct gene transfer into mouse muscle *in vivo*. *Science* 1990; **247**: 1465–8

11 Russell SJ, Hawkins RE, Winter G. Retroviral vectors displaying functional antibody fragments. *Nucl Acids Res* 1993; **21**: 1081–5

12 Hawkins RE, Winter G, Hamblin TJ, Stevenson FK, Russell SJ. A genetic approach to anti-idiotype immunisation. *J Immunother* 1993; **14**: 272–8

13 Ulmer JB, Donnelly JJ, Parker SE, *et al*. Heterologous protection against influenza by injection of DNA encoding a viral protein. *Science* 1993; **259**: 1745–9

14 Watanabe A, Raz E, Kohsaka H, *et al*. Induction of antibodies to a k V region by gene immunisation. *J Immunol* 1993; **151**: 2871–6

Anti-idiotype vaccine in colorectal cancer

Lindy Durrant

CRC Department of Clinical Oncology, University of Nottingham, City Hospital, Hucknall Road, Nottingham, UK

A human monoclonal anti-idiotypic antibody, 105AD7, which mimics a colorectal tumour associated antigen, 791Tgp72, has been developed [1]. 105AD7 induced DTH responses to 791Tgp72 positive human tumour cells in mice and rats [2], and was therefore a candidate immunogen for idiotypic immunotherapy of colorectal cancer patients. Phase I clinical studies in advanced colorectal cancer patients showed that immunisation with 105AD7 is non-toxic. Immunised patients showed evidence of T-cell blastogenesis responses to 791Tgp72 expressing cells and enhanced IL-2 production [3]; antibody to 105AD7 or tumour has not been detected. Moreover patients in the 105AD7 study had a brisk and significant lymphocytosis following immunisation.

Notably, 105AD7 immunised patients had increased survival when compared with a contemporary group of patients treated in the same centre [4]. These encouraging results are currently being confirmed in a double blind randomised study in a similar cohort of patients under the auspices of the CRC Phase I/II committee.

Several T-cell mechanisms could account for the apparent delayed progression of tumour growth after 105AD7 immunisation. These included specific and non specific activation of MHC restricted regulatory and effector T-cells and T-cell recruitment and activation of other non-specific effect or mechanisms. These issues are being addressed in a clinical study in which primary colorectal cancer patients are immunised pre-operatively, and responses analysed peri-operatively.

Cytotoxicity against autologous tumour cells was studied in six patients with rectal cancer immunised pre-operatively with 105AD7. Peripheral blood lymphocytes taken prior to immunisation were tested against tumour cells extracted from biopsies also obtained prior to immunisation or natural killer (NK) sensitive target cells. Cryopreserved lymphocytes taken before and after tumour immunisation, fresh peripheral blood lymphocytes taken immediately prior to surgery and lymphocytes from tumour draining lymph nodes were tested against autologous cells from the resected specimen or NK sensitive targets. Significant killing of autologous tumour cells which was not due to NK activity was seen with cryopreserved lymphocytes or lymph node cells of three patients at 1–2 weeks post immunisation with 105AD7 but not on pretreatment biopsies. Enhanced NK activity was seen 2–3 weeks post immunisation in 3/6 patients. These results indicate that 105AD7 human monoclonal antibody immunisation enhances cytotoxicity in rectal cancer patients by specific and non-specific effector mechanisms [5].

Thus treatment of rectal cancer patients by injection of the human monoclonal anti-idiotypic antibody produced a time dependent killing of autologous tumour cells in three patients which appears to be unrelated to NK activity. The main cytolytic effector cells of the immune system are CD8 expressing cytotoxic T-lymphocytes that recognise via their specific T-cell receptors, antigenic peptides of eight or nine amino acids complexed with major histocompatibility complex (MHC) class I molecules on the surface of target cells. Other accessory and adhesion molecules as well as cytokines are also necessary for the expression of efficient cytotoxicity. It is unclear at present whether the killing of autologous tumour cells in 105AD7 immunised patients is a result of clonal expansion of specific cytotoxic T-cells but in this context analysis of T-cell subsets in the peripheral blood of immunised patients showed a decrease in the ratio of CD8 RA/RO cells suggesting activated T killer cells were accumulating following immunisation with 105AD7.

Class I MHC molecules conventionally present endogenously synthesised antigens whereas exogenous protein antigens enter the class II presentation pathway. However, a subset of antigen presenting cells has been shown to process and present extracellular antigens to stimulate MHC class I restricted responses. Similarly protein antigens incorporated into immunostimulating complexes or encapsulated into certain liposomes can stimulate CTL immunity. The human anti-idiotypic monoclonal antibody may also be presented in the context of MHC class I by one of these mechanisms.

The anti-idiotypic antibody could be stimulating CD4 helper T-cells which facilitate activation of pre-existing but silent anti-tumour cytotoxic T-cells. Our initial phase I studies showed elevated levels of serum IL-2 associated with 105AD7 immunisation. Activation of helper T-cells could also explain the enhanced NK activity seen post 105AD7 immunisation in 3/6 of the rectal cancer patients. Human NK cells could be direct effectors against tumour cells, together with T-cell they could produce cytokines such as IFN-gamma, TNF-alpha, granulocyte-macrophage colony stimulating factor, some of which may enhance anti-tumour activity from other endogenous lytic effectors or act by a combination of direct and indirect mechanisms.

The requirement for T-cell help for CTL induction particularly *in vivo* suggests that the anti-idiotypic antibody could contain both CD4 helper and CD8 CTL epitopes. In this context it has been shown that determinant linkage of helper and CTL epitopes is the basis for productive interaction between the two T-cells and the same antigen presenting cell, and that IL-2 and IFN-gamma play a crucial role

The peri-operative study in rectal cancer patients has now been extended to colonic patients and recruitment of inflammatory cells at the tumour site is being studied by immunocytochemistry. The number of infiltrating cells within the tumour of immunised patients is being quantified on serial sections from different sites within a tumour by image analysis using the NIH IMAGE program. The number of inflammatory cells within the tumours of 105AD7 immunised patients will be compared to the number of cells infiltrating tumours of immunised patients. Early results indicate an increase in the numbers of activated CD4+ T-cells and NK cells. The latter is of particular interest as NK cells are rarely found in colorectal tumours.

There is accumulating evidence in colorectal cancer patients that 105AD7 presents a multiplex of T-cell epitopes. A better understanding of which of these are essential for the generation of protective anti-tumour immunity will underpin the development of new therapeutic vaccines for cancer.

REFERENCES

1 Austin EB, Robins RA, Durrant LG, Price MR, Baldwin RW. Human monoclonal anti-idiotypic antibody to the tumour associated antibody 791T/36. *Immunology* 1989; **67**: 525–30

2 Austin EB, Robins RA, Baldwin RW, Durrant LG. Induction of delayed hypersensitivity to human tumour cells with a human monoclonal anti idiotypic antibody. *J Natl Cancer Inst* 1991; **83**: 1245–8

3 Robins RA, Denton GWL, Hardcastle JD, Austin EB, Baldwin RW, Durrant LG. Anti-tumour immune response and Interleukin 2 production induced in colorectal cancer patients by immunisation with human monoclonal anti-idiotypic antibody. *Cancer Res* 1991; **51**: 5425–9

4 Denton GWL, Durrant LG, Hardcastle JD, Austin EB, Sewell HF, Robins RA. Clinical outcome of colorectal cancer patients treated with human monoclonal anti-idiotypic antibody. *Int J Cancer* 1994; **57**: 10–4

5 Durrant LG, Buckley D, Denton GWL, Hardcastle JD, Sewell HF, Robins RA. Enhanced cell mediated tumour killing in patients immunised with human monoclonal anti-idiotypic antibody 105AD7. *Cancer Res* 1994; **54**: 4837–40

Immunotherapy with antibody-cytokine fusion proteins

Ralph A. Reisfeld

The Scripps Research Institute, N. Torrey Pines Road, La Jolla, CA, USA

The application of recombinant DNA technology has recently led to the construction of antibody-cytokine fusion proteins, designed to achieve optimal biological effectiveness by combining the unique targeting ability of antibodies with the multifunctional activities of cytokines [1–3]. Antibody-cytokine fusion proteins have been proposed for the treatment of solid tumours, including melanoma [2] and carcinoma [4,5].

Here, we evaluated a genetically engineered fusion protein, ch14.18-IL-2, consisting of chimeric anti-ganglioside GD2 antibody (ch14.18) and recombinant human interleukin 2 (rhIL-2) for its ability to suppress dissemination and growth of human neuroblastoma in a pre-clinical model. After submission of this manuscript, a paper appeared that describes in detail the data summarized here (H. Sabzevari *et al. Proc Natl Acad Sci USA* 1994; **91**: 9626–30). The ch14.18-IL-2 fusion protein was shown previously to target IL-2 to tumour cells and to stimulate T cell-mediated killing of autologous melanoma cells *in vitro* [2]. In addition, prior clinical studies indicated that prolonged, partial and complete remissions of paediatric neuroblastoma could be induced by both murine anti-GD2 antibody 14.G2a [6] and its human/chimeric variant ch14.18 [7]. Therapy of neuroblastoma patients with rhIL-2 and mAb 14.G2a also generated conditions within the peripheral blood of these patients that enabled their own lymphocytes to mediate antibody-dependent cellular cytotoxicity (ADCC) sufficiently to effectively kill human neuroblastoma cells *in vitro* [9]. Taken together, these findings provided a rationale for evaluating the efficacy of an anti-GD2-IL-2 fusion protein in killing human neuroblastoma cells *in vivo*.

Our primary aim was to test the hypothesis that this fusion protein can specifically target rhIL-2 to tumour sites and is more effective than rhIL-2 in achieving efficient tumour cell lysis. We could demonstrate that this was the case in an adoptive immunotherapy model for experimental hepatic metastasis of human neuroblastoma in SCID mice reconstituted with human lymphokine-activated killer (LAK) cells. Specifically, one day after intrasplenic injection of 5×10^5 SK-N-AS neuroblastoma cells and induction of hepatic metastasis, a control group received daily i.p. injections of 0.2 ml PBS. The other animals were each injected i.p. with 4×10^7 human LAK cells and then randomised into experimental groups, each being injected i.p. for seven days with one of the following: 0.2 ml PBS; ch14.18; ch14.18 plus rhIL-2 or ch14.18-IL-2 fusion protein containing an equivalent amount of rhIL-2. When animals were sacrificed and livers examined for neuroblastoma metastases, one month after tumour cell injection, there was a lack of a statistically significant difference from controls in the number of hepatic metastases found in SCID mice treated with either PBS or LAK cells. Most of these animals presented with a very large number (>500) of metastatic foci in their livers and exhibited up to three-fold greater liver weights than untreated animals. Although SCID mice treated with LAK cells plus ch14.18 showed a statistical significant decrease ($p=0.01$) in the number of metastatic foci, all of these animals presented with metastases ranging from five to 100 liver foci and had increased liver weights. In contrast, all SCID mice treated with the ch14.18-IL-2 fusion protein revealed a complete absence of macroscopic metastatic liver foci ($p=0.003$) and also presented with normal liver weights. However, when SCID mice were treated with a mixture of ch14.18 and rhIL-2 at dose levels equivalent to the ch14.18-IL-2 fusion protein, they also showed a complete lack of macroscopic metastatic liver foci.

Identical results were obtained when SCID mice were treated with high doses (7.5×10^5 IU/day) of rhIL-2, *per se*. Since we observed these same effects with both ch14.18-IL-2 and a mixture of ch14.18 and rhIL-2 at these relatively high dose levels, i.e. 250 μg ch14.18-IL-2, we compared their effect at lower dose levels. Surprisingly, we found that as little as 1 μg of ch14.18-IL-2 per injection proved effective in suppressing dissemination and growth of metastasis. Indeed, dose levels of 1, 8 and 16 μg of ch14.18-IL-2 fusion protein were far more capable in suppressing growth of tumour metastasis than equivalent doses of rhIL-2. Moreover, another set of experiments indicated that relatively low dose levels of ch14.18-IL-2 (1 and 16 μg) were also more proficient than equivalent amounts of rhIL-2 (3,000 and 48,000 IU) in prolonging the life span of tumour bearing SCID mice reconstituted with human LAK cells.

The choice of our adoptive immunotherapy model in SCID mice reconstituted with human LAK cells was based on the following considerations. First, the model was highly reproducible, as hepatic metastases were routinely found in 100% of the SCID mice four weeks post intrasplenic injection of human neuroblastoma cells. Second, LAK cells were easily and reproducibly available in large numbers by stimulation of human PBMCs with rhIL-2 and up to 20% of LAK cells were detected in the liver of SCID mice 48 h after i.p. injection. In this regard, human LAK cells were reported to remain viable in the liver of SCID mice for up to 14 days [8]. Third, a further rationale for using LAK cells in our model is that treatment of paediatric neuroblastoma patients with IL-2 plus mAb 14.G2a was reported to induce effector cells capable of mediating LAK activity against NK resistant Daudi target cells and that further IL-2 treatment of these LAK cells greatly enhanced their cytolytic activity against neuroblastoma cells [8].

Although we found that in our experimental model the ch14.18-IL-2 protein effectively activated human LAK cells to suppress neuroblastoma dissemination and growth, the ability of recombinant antibody-IL-2 fusion proteins to activate effector cells is by no means limited to LAK cells. Thus, treatment of neuroblastoma patients with anti-GD2 antibody plus rhIL-2 induced ADCC of the patients' peripheral blood mononuclear cells sufficient to effectively kill neuroblastoma cells *in vitro* [8]. In preclinical studies of human melanoma, we also found that antibody-IL-2 fusion proteins can activate tumour infiltrating lymphocytes (2), as well as other leukocytes bearing FcγRIII and/or high affinity IL-2 receptors, including natural killer cells and CD8+ activated T-cells [10].

We clearly established that a high dose (250 μg/injection) of ch14.18-IL-2 is more effective than either LAK cells or LAK cells+ch14.18 in suppressing growth of human neuroblastoma metastasis in SCID mice. However, it was particularly impressive that the fusion protein can achieve this effect at very low dose levels (1 μg/injection) and more effectively than equivalent amounts of rhIL-2. These findings are encouraging for two reasons. First, they strongly support our hypothesis that recombinant antibody-cytokine fusion proteins can specifically target cytokines to tumour sites and stimulate immune effector cells sufficiently to achieve efficient tumour cell lysis. Second, the fact that very low dose levels of the ch14.18-IL-2 fusion protein proved more effective than equivalent amounts of rhIL-2 in suppressing tumour growth in SCID mice and in prolonging their life span suggests that it may also be feasible to apply an optimal biological dose of ch14.18-IL-2 for future treatment of paediatric neuroblastoma patients. Third, based on our data, one might anticipate that the potentially lower effective dose levels of ch14.18-IL-2 may produce less toxicity than the relatively high dose levels of rhIL-2 necessary to achieve anti-tumour effects in clinical applications.

In summary, we demonstrated here that the ch14.18-IL-2 fusion protein can effectively suppress dissemination and growth of hepatic metastasis of human neuroblastoma in SCID mice reconstituted with human LAK cells. This antibody-cytokine fusion protein was shown to be superior in this regard to an equivalent dose of rhIL-2 and also proved more capable in prolonging the life span of these animals. Although we realise the limitations of our experimental metastasis model in SCID mice in terms of its predictive value for the eventual clinical effectiveness of ch14.18-IL-2, we believe that this recombinant fusion protein may hold some promise for future treatment of human neuroblastoma and other GD2-expressing tumours in an adjuvant setting.

REFERENCES

1 Gillies SD, Young D, Lo K-M, Foley SF, Reisfeld RA. Expression of genetically engineered immunoconjugates of lymphotoxin and a chimeric anti-ganglioside GD2 antibody. *Hybridoma* 1991; **10**: 347–56

2 Gillies SD, Reilly EB, Lo K-M, Reisfeld RA. Antibody-targeted interleukin 2 stimulates T-cell killing of autologous tumor cells. *Proc Natl Acad Sci USA* 1992; **89**: 1428–32

3 Gillies SD, Young D, Lo K-M, Roberts S. Biological activity and *in vivo* clearance of antitumor antibody/cytokine fusion proteins. *Bioconjugate Chem* 1993; **4**: 230–35

4 Gillies SD, Wesolowski JS, Lo K-M. Targeting human cytotoxic T lymphocytes to kill heterologous epidermal growth factor receptor-bearing tumor cells. *J Immunol* 1990; **146**: 1067–71

5 Fell HP, Gayle MA, Grosmaire L, Ledbetter JA. Genetic construction and characterization of a fusion protein consisting of a chimeric F(ab′) with specificity for carcinomas and human IL-2. *J Immunol* 1991; **146**: 2446–52

6 Handgretinger R, Baader P, Dopfer R *et al*. A phase I study of neuroblastoma with the anti-ganglioside GD2 antibody 14.G2a. *Cancer Immunol Immunother* 1992; **35**: 199–204

7 Handgretinger R, Anderson K, Dopfer R *et al*. A phase I study of human/mouse chimeric antiganglioside GD2 antibody

ch14.18 in patients with neuroblastoma. *Eur J Cancer* 1994; (in press)

8 Hank JA, Surfus J, Gan J *et al*. Treatment of neuroblastoma patients with antiganglioside GD2 antibody plus interleukin-2 induces antibody-dependent cellular cytotoxicity against neuroblastoma detected *in vitro*. *J Immunother* 1994; **15**: 29–37

9 Takahashi H, Nakada T, Puisieux I. Inhibition of human colon cancer growth by antibody-directed human LAK cells in SCID mice. *Science* 1993; **259**: 1460–3

10 Naramura M, Gillies SD, Mendelsohn J, Reisfeld RA, Mueller BM. Mechanisms of cellular cytotoxicity mediated by a recombinant antibody-IL-2 fusion protein against human melanoma cells. *Immunol Letters* 1994; **39**: 91–9

The human response to therapeutic antibodies

Jonathan A. Ledermann
Department of Oncology, University College London Medical School, London, UK

It has become clear that most patients will develop anti-antibodies following administration of mouse monoclonal antibodies for diagnostic or therapeutic purposes. In some patients a human anti-mouse antibody (HAMA) response appears after a single diagnostic dose of monoclonal antibody, whilst in others repeated doses of therapeutic antibody may be given before HAMA appears. The reasons for the variablity are not fully understood but they probably depend on host factors as well as the intrinsic immunogenicity of the antibody. HAMA usually appears 10-30 days after exposure and in its presence further administration of antitumour antibody leads to the formation of immune complexes and rapid clearance of therapeutic antibodies from the circulation into the liver and spleen, preventing the anti-tumour antibody from reaching its target. The altered pharmacokinetics of the monoclonal antibody are often accompanied by acute allergic manifestations in the patient. The success of immunoconjugate therapy depends on the ability to use antibodies repeatedly as vehicles to carry cytotoxic compounds such as radiopharmaceuticals, immunotoxins or enzymes to tumours. The formation of HAMA has a detrimental effect on immunoconjugate therapy and it needs to be prevented.

It is known that patients with B-cell lymphoma are less likely to develop HAMA than patients receiving treatment for solid cancers, probably because they are immuno-suppressed. Several strategies have been developed to prevent allograft rejection using drugs such as azathioprine, cyclophosphamide, prednisolone and cyclosporin A. Cell-mediated immunity is most successfully suppressed by cyclosporin A but this drug also inhibits humoral immunity. Some years ago we investigated the action of cyclosporin A on the formation of anti-antibodies in animals challenged with mouse monclonal antibodies. Studies in rabbits

indicated that intramuscular injection of cyclosporin A suppressed the immune response to two courses of anti-tumour antibodies. Some animals developed prolonged immunosuppression and failed to respond to further challenge with antibody [1]. In a clinical trial of therapy with ^{131}I A5B7, an IgG$_1$ mouse monoclonal antibody to carcinoembryonic antigen cyclosporin A was given to suppress the HAMA response. Therapeutic doses of antibody were given every two weeks and oral cyclosporin A, 24 mg/kg, was given daily for six days starting 48 h before the first therapeutic dose of antibody. Cyclosporin A delayed the formation of HAMA and attenuated the immune response. Up to four courses of ^{131}I A5B7 were given over a period of two months but in the absence of cyclosporin A all patients developed HAMA after two doses of antibody [2]. The high dose cyclosporin A produced considerable nausea and in subsequent studies cyclosporin A, given continuously at 15 mg/kg/d produced fewer gastrointestinal side effects without compromising its immunosuppressive effect [3]. Tumour targeting and the pharmacokinetics of ^{131}I A5B7 were unchanged even in the presence of small quantities of HAMA provided that cyclosporin A was continued. Further therapy was limited by myelotoxicity from the radiopharmaceutical. Drugs such as cyclophos-phamide, prednisolone and azathioprine have also been used but they have had little effect on the HAMA response.

Many patients have 'pre-existing' antibodies reactive with mouse antibody. These appear to be rheumatoid-like factors and they do not interfere with initial monoclonal antibody therapy. Immune responses are most frequently directed against the mouse constant region of the immunoglobulin molecule although anti-idiotypic binding is also seen, particularly after frequent exposure to mouse antibody [4,5]. It may therefore by possible to reduce the immunogenicity of an antibody by removing the Fc portion of the molecule, masking its immunogenic sites, or by producing a 'humanised' antibody. In uncontrolled studies it appears that therapy with Fab' fragments is less likely to elicit an antiglobulin response. However, the small size and short half life of Fab' fragments may make their use less desirable as therapeutic agents, and anti-idiotypic immunisation may occur. Encouraging preclinical results have been reported using chemically modified immunoglobulin to prevent immunisation to intact IgG. These include attachment of polyethylene glycol to antibody to make it less immunogenic [6] or conjugation to daunomycin leading to cytotoxic clonal elimination of reactive B-cells [7]. The latter is an attractive approach which probably depends critically on how the cytotoxic agent is processed by immune cells as it does not operate in man when radiolabelled antibody is used.

Waldman *et al.* [8] have established animal models to induce tolerance using anti T-cell antibodies. Recent trials with humanised antibodies have shown that some autoimmune diseases can be modified in man. The mechanism of action of these antibodies is not yet fully understood but this approach might in the future be used to prevent an immune response to immunoconjugates.

Improvements in recombinant DNA technology have largely replaced efforts to produce human monoclonal antibodies. It is now possible to produce human-mouse chimeric antibodies with mouse variable regions inserted into a human framework, or more specific 'humanised' antibodies where only the mouse cdr regions are used. Some of these engineered molecules have entered clinical trials and the most detailed information comes from studies with two antibodies; chimeric B72.3, an humanised IgG$_4$ antibody reacting with the TAG-72 antigen, a high molecular weight mucin, and chimeric 17-1A, an IgG$_1$ that recognises a widely distributed epithelial surface antigen. Our own work and that of LoBuglio's group have shown that chimeric B72.3 with mouse V-regions joined to a human gamma-4 framework remains immunogenic. We found that five out of 14 patients were immunised after one course of mouse/human ^{131}I B72.3. In patients who did not develop an anti-antibody response therapy could be repeated up to five times at 3–4 week intervals. LoBuglio's group [9] reported immune responses in seven out of 12 patients after an initial infusion of chimeric B72.3. Thus, this mouse/human chimeric antibody is only slightly less immunogenic than murine B72.3 which leads to a HAMA response in over 70% of patients after a single injection. The immune response is directed against mouse V regions but in some cases anti-antibodies react with novel epitopes

at the junction of the V-region and human framework (CH1). These results contrast strikingly with those from studies with chimeric 17-1 where only one out of 10 patients developed an immune response [10]. Genetically engineered antibody fragments produced in bacteria are now being prepared for clinical trials. These small molecules are least likely to be immunogenic but the possibility of anti-idiotypic immunisation still exists.

Therapy with unconjugated antibody has had a chequered history but tumour responses do undoubtedly occur. Most responses are short-lived but reports of a sustained response to anti-idiotype therapy in B-cell lymphoma and improved survival of colorectal cancer patients with adjuvant antibody therapy provides a source of encouragement [11,12]. In the recently reported trial of adjuvant 17-1A therapy in colorectal cancer 80% of patients developed HAMA responses by the second or third infusion. Such responses did not appear to influence the probability of patients remaining disease-free. There is also some evidence to suggest that patients with metastatic colorectal cancer who make an anti-idiotypic (AB2) response fare better [13]. AB3 responses to AB2 have been demonstrated in patients and the results of preliminary trials with anti-idiotypic immunisation are encouraging [14–16]. However, it is unclear whether anti-tumour activity is due to modulation of the idiotypic network as both humoral and proliferative T-cell responses are detectable [17].

In summary, anti-antibody responses do not appear to affect adversely the results of therapy with unconjugated antibody; on the contrary they may be beneficial and anti-idiotype therapy is an active area of investigation. This contrasts with the need to prevent humoral responses to immunoconjugates and genetically engineered humanised antibodies provide an obvious way forward. However, toxins or enzymes conjugated to these molecules remain immunogenic and immunosuppression strategies are still likely to be required.

REFERENCES

1 Ledermann JA, Begent RHJ, Bagshawe KD. Cyclosporin A prevents the anti-murine antibody response to a monoclonal antibody in rabbits. *Br J Cancer* 1988; **58**: 562–6

2 Ledermann JA, Begent RHJ, Bagshawe KD, *et al.* Repeated antitumour antibody therapy in man with suppression of the host response by cyclosporin A. *Br J Cancer* 1988; **58**: 654-7

3 Ledermann JA, Begent RHJ, Massof C, Kelly AMB, Adam T, Bagshawe KD. A phase I study of repeated therapy with

radiolabelled antibody to carcinoembryonic antigen using intermittent or continuous administration of cyclosporin A to suppress the immune response. *Int J Cancer* 1991; **47**: 659–64

4 Courtenay-Luck NS, Epenetos AA, Moore R, *et al*. Development of primary and secondary immune responses to mouse monoclonal antibodies used in the diagnosis and therapy of malignant neoplasms. *Cancer Res* 1986; **46**: 6489–93

5 Courtenay-Luck NS, Epenetos AA, Winearls CG, Ritter MA. Pre-existing human anti-murine immunoglobulin reactivity due to polyclonal rheumatoid factors. *Cancer Res* 1987; **47**: 4520–5

6 Wilkinson I, Jackson C-JC, Lang GM, Holdford-Strevens V, Sehon AH. Tolerance induction in mice by conjugates of monoclonal immunoglobulins and monomethoxypolyethylene glycol. *J Immunol* 1987; **139**: 326–31

7 Durrant LG, Robins AR, Marksman RA, Garnett MC, Ogunmuyiwa Y, Baldwin RW. Abrogation of antibody responses in rats to murine monoclonal antibody 791T/36 by treatment with daunomycin-cis-aconityl 791T/36 conjugates. *Cancer Immunol Immunother* 1989; **28**: 37–43

8 Waldmann H, Cobbold S. The use of monoclonal antibodies to achieve immunological tolerance. *Immunol Today* 1993; **14**(6): 247–51

9 Khazeli MB, Saleh MN, Liu TP, *et al*. Pharmacokinetics and immune response of 131I- chimeric mouse/human B72.3 (human γ4) monoclonal antibody in humans. *Cancer Res* 1991; **51**: 5461–6

10 LoBuglio AF, Wheeler RH, Trang J, *et al*. Mouse/human chimeric monoclonal antibody in man: kinetics and immune response. *Proc Natl Acad Sci USA* 1989; **86**: 4220–4

11 Miller RA, Maloney DG, Warnke R, Levy R. Treatment of B cell lymphoma with a monoclonal anti-idiotype antibody. *N Engl J Med* 1982; **306**: 517–22

12 Reithmüller G, Schneider-Gädicke E, Schlimok G, *et al*. Randomised trial of monoclonal antibody for adjuvant therapy of resected Duke's C colorectal carcinoma. *Lancet* 1994; **i**: 1177–83

13 Koprowski H, Herlyn D, Lubeck M, DeFreitas E, Sears HF. Human anti-idiotype antibodies in cancer patients: Is the modulation of the immune response beneficial for the patient? *Proc Natl Acad Sci USA* 1984; **81**: 216–19

14 Herlyn D, Caton A, Koprowski H. Anti-idiotypes in cancer immunotherapy. In: Epenetos A, ed. *Monclonal antibodies applications in clinical oncology*. London: Chapman & Hall, 1991: 283–290

15 Durrant LG, Denton GW, Jacobs E, *et al*. An idiotypic replica of carcinoembryonic antigen inducing cellular and humoral responses directed against human colorectal tumours. *Int J Cancer* 1992; **50**(5): 811–16

16 Denton GW, Durrant LG, Hardcastle JD, Austin EB, Sewell HF, Robins RA. Clinical outcome of colorectal cancer patients treated with human monoclonal anti-idiotypic antibody. *Int J Cancer* 1994; **57**(1): 10–14

17 Kwak LW, Campbell MJ, Czerwinski DK, Hart S, Miller RA, Levy R. Induction of responses in patients with B-cell lymphoma against the surface-immuoglobulin idiotype expressed by their tumours. *N Engl J Med* 1992; **327**: 1209–15

ADEPT—principles and experimental studies

Surinder K. Sharma

CRC Clinical Research Laboratories, Department of Clinical Oncology, Royal Free Hospital School of Medicine, London, UK

Monoclonal antibodies directed at human tumour associated antigens, directly conjugated to radioisotopes, drugs and toxins, have been used to achieve a relatively selective killing of tumour cells without much systemic toxicity. However the limited success of this system has been due to the heterogeneity of antigen expression by the tumour cells and the fact that most of the cytotoxic agents require internalisation by the cell to exert their toxic effect. The uptake of a radiolabelled antibody by cells may be directly proportional to the antigen density at the cell surface with the result that the antibody-isotope conjugate would target to cells with high antigen content and any cell not expressing the antigen would only be killed by the cross-fire effect if they were in close proximity of the radiation pathway of the isotope. Cells exposed to sublethal doses may survive by antigenic modulation and lack antigen expression so that selective killing of antigen expressing cells would only tend to increase resistant populations.

The ADEPT or antibody directed enzyme prodrug therapy approach has been designed to overcome some of these limitations. In the ADEPT system [1–3], antibodies directed at human tumour associated antigens are used to target enzymes to tumours. After enzyme has been cleared from blood and other non-tumour sites, a prodrug, which is matched to the enzyme, is given. The enzyme converts the relatively non-toxic prodrug into a cytotoxic drug at the tumour sites. The drug formed is designed to diffuse into nearby cells, some of which may be antigen negative. The ADEPT system has the advantage that the enzyme may act as an amplification system with each enzyme molecule catalysing many molecules of prodrug. Several other workers have studied similar approaches [4–8].

In our studies with ADEPT, we have used F(ab′)2 fragments of monoclonal antibodies (W14 and SB10)

directed at human chorionic gonadotrophin (hCG) and A5B7 directed at carcinoembryonic antigen (CEA). These have been chemically conjugated via a stable thioether bond [9] to a bacterial enzyme carboxypeptidase G2 (CPG2) which catalyses the hydrolytic cleavage of reduced and non-reduced folates. The catalytic activity of native and conjugated CPG2 was measured by a spectrophotometric assay using methotrexate as a substrate.

The ADEPT system has been studied in a human choriocarcinoma (CC3) xenograft as a two phase system with complete eradication of a high proportion of tumours with only one ADEPT cycle [3,10] and in a human colon carcinoma xenograft (LS174T) resulting in a growth delay of the tumour [11]. ADEPT three phase studies previously carried out in the LS174T xenograft [2,12] have been extended to a CEA expressing human ovarian carcinoma xenograft (OvCa) [13].

As the targeting of enzymes to tumours is dependent on pharmacokinetics and biodistribution of the antibody to which it is conjugated, it is therefore influenced by such factors as nature of antigen to be targeted, intact antibody or fragments, conjugation methods and size of the tumours. Biodistribution studies with radiolabelled A5B7-F(ab′)2-CPG2 showed these to localise optimally within 24 h in both LS174T and OvCa xenografts. The conjugate cleared from blood over a period of time by which time the enzyme levels in the tumours were less than those at 24 h. Therefore to optimise use of localised conjugate, it may be desirable to accelerate the clearance of enzyme activity from plasma after tumour localisation has occurred. High levels of enzyme activity in plasma and non-specific retention of conjugate in normal tissues may result in prodrug activation in these sites. Therefore, some form of enzyme inactivation or accelerated clearance mechanism may be employed to minimise toxicity in the normal tissues. We have studied two methods in which accelerated clearance of residual CPG2 may be achieved. The first method involves a monoclonal anti-CPG2 antibody (SB43) which inactivates CPG2 *in vitro* and *in vivo* [14]. To avoid potential inactivation of CPG2 at the tumour sites, SB43 was galactosylated [15] which allowed inactivation and clearance of the conjugate from blood via carbohydrate receptors in the liver [16] without affecting tumour localisation of the conjugate. The second method involved galactosylation of the conjugate such that it cleared rapidly from blood. To allow localisation of the conjugate, an inhibitor [17] which binds competitively to the asialoglycoprotein receptor, was injected. This maintained high blood levels of the conjugate for a period of time to allow tumour localisation, followed by rapid clearance of the conjugate from blood [18]. Experimental therapy studies, in LS174T xenografts, using both clearance mechanisms gave similar growth delay of the tumours. Alternative to SB43gal would be an antibody which does not inactivate the enzyme but would bind to other epitopes on the conjugate. Also use of anti-idiotypic antibodies to accelerate the conjugate may be another option. Use of steptavidin/biotin clearance system [19] in combination with galactosylation procedures may also be explored in ADEPT.

Experimental therapy studies in both LS174T and OvCa xenografts were carried out using a three phase ADEPT system in which the first phase consisted of localisation of conjugate at tumour sites followed at 20 h by an injection of SB43gal to inactivate and clear residual enzyme from blood. The prodrug, CMDA, was given as the third phase. These studies with one ADEPT cycle only have shown a consistent and reproducible growth delay of the tumours compared to the control either untreated or treated with CPG2 conjugated to a non-specific antibody, the prodrug alone or repeated treatment with some of the conventional chemotherapeutic agents. With the CMDA prodrug, repeated ADEPT cycles may be necessary to maintain growth delay in these models. However as murine monoclonal antibodies have been used to target a bacterial enzyme to tumours, both components of the conjugate are potentially immunogenic in the human. Our studies carried out in normal Balb/C mice showed the presence of anti-CPG2 antibodies in mouse blood within 10 days after a single injection of the conjugate [20]. In the pilot clinical trial of ADEPT, a number of patients given one dose of conjugate developed immune response to both the murine antibody (HAMA) and CPG2 within 10 days of the conjugate

infusion [21]. However using immunosuppressive agents such as cyclosporin A in subsequent patients it was possible to extend treatment to more than one cycle of ADEPT. The first clinical trial of ADEPT [22] in patients with advanced colorectal cancer has shown feasibility of this approach as a treatment for cancer.

Acknowledgment

This work was funded by the Cancer Research Campaign. These studies were carried out in collaboration with Professor K. D. Bagshawe, Dr P. J. Burke, Dr G. T. Rogers, Dr C. J. Springer and J. A. Boden.

REFERENCES

1 Bagshawe KD. Antibody directed enzymes revive anti-cancer prodrugs concept. *Br J Cancer* 1987; **56**: 531–2
2 Bagshawe KD. Towards generating cytotoxic agents at cancer sites. *Br J Cancer* 1989; **60**: 275–81
3 Bagshawe KD, Springer CJ, Searle F, *et al.* A cytotoxic agent can be generated selectively at cancer sites. *Br J Cancer* 1988; **58**: 700–3
4 Senter PD, Saulnier MG, Schreiber GH *et al.* Anti-tumour effects of antibody-alkaline phosphatase conjugates in combination with etoposide phosphate. *Proc Natl Acad Sci USA* 1988; **85**: 4842–6
5 Senter PD, Schreiber GH, Hirschberg DL *et al.* Enhancement of the *in-vitro* and *in-vivo* antitumour activities of phosphorylated mitomycin C and etoposide derivatives by monoclonal antibody-alkaline phosphatase conjugates. *Cancer Res* 1989; **49**: 5789–92
6 Bosslet K, Czech J, Lorenz P, Sedlack HH, Schuermann M, Seemann G. Molecular and functional characterisation of a fusion protein suited for tumour specific prodrug activation. *Br J Cancer* 1992; **65**: 234–8
7 Meyer DL, Jungheim LN, Law KL, *et al.* Site-specific prodrug activation by antibody-beta-lactamase conjugates: Regression and long-term growth inhibition of human colon carcinoma xenograft models. *Cancer Res* 1993; **53**: 3956–63
8 Wallace PM, MacMaster JF, Smith VF *et al.* Intratumour generation of 5-Fluorouracil mediated by an antibody-cytosine deaminase conjugate in combination with 5-Fluorocytosine. *Cancer Res* 1994; **54**: 2719–23
9 Melton RG, Boyle JMB, Rogers GT *et al.* Optimisation of small scale coupling of A5B7 monoclonal antibody to carboxypeptidase G2. *J Immunol Methods* 1993; **158**: 49–56
10 Springer CJ, Bagshawe KD, Sharma SK *et al.* Ablation of human choriocarcinoma xenografts in nude mice by antibody

directed enzyme prodrug therapy (ADEPT) with three novel compounds. *Eur J Cancer* 1991; **27**: 1361–6

11 Blakey DC, Valcaccia BE, East S, *et al.* Anti-tumour effects of an antibody carboxydase G2 conjugate in combination with a benzoic acid mustard prodrug. *Cell Biophysics* 1993; **22**: 1–8

12 Sharma SK, Bagshawe KD, Springer CJ, *et al.* Antibody directed enzyme prodrug therapy (ADEPT): A three phase system. *Disease Markers* 1991; **9**: 225–31

13 Sharma SK, Boden JA, Springer CJ, Burke PJ, Bagshawe KD. ADEPT studies in human ovarian carcinoma xenografts. In press

14 Sharma SK, Bagshawe KD, Burke PJ, Boden RW, Rogers GT. Inactivation and clearance of an anti-CEA carboxypeptidase G2 conjugate in blood after localisation in a xenograft model. *Br J Cancer* 1990; **61**: 659–62

15 Mattes MJ. Biodistribution of antibodies after intraperitoneal or intravenous injection and effect of carbohydrate modifications. *J Natl Cancer Inst* 1987; **79**: 855–63

16 Thornburg RW, Day JF, Baynes JW, Thorpe SR. Carbohydrate mediated clearance of immune complexes from circulation: a role for galactose residues in the hepatic uptake of IgG-antigen complexes. *J Biol Chem* 1980; **255**: 6820–5

17 Ong GL, Ettenson D, Sharkey RM *et al.* Galactose conjugated antibodies in cancer therapy: Properties and principles of action. *Cancer Res* 1991; **51**: 1619–26

18 Sharma SK, Bagshawe KD, Burke PJ, *et al.* Galactosylated antibodies and antibody-enzyme conjugates in antibody directed enzyme prodrug therapy. *Cancer*, 1994: **73**: 1114–20

19 Marshall D, Pedley RB, Melton RG *et al.* Galactosylated streptavidin for improved clearance of biotinylated intact and F(ab′)2 fragments of an anti-tumour antibody. *Br J Cancer* 1995; in press

20 Sharma SK, Bagshawe KD, Melton RG, Sherwood RF. Immunogenicity of antibody-enzyme conjugates in antibody directed enzyme prodrug therapy (ADEPT). *Antibody, Immunoconj Radiopharm* 1991; **4**: 226

21 Sharma SK, Bagshawe KD, Melton RG, Sherwood RF. Human immune response to monoclonal antibody-enzyme conjugates in ADEPT pilot clinical trial. *Cell Biophysics* 1993; **23**: 109–20

22 Bagshawe KD, Sharma SK, Springer CJ *et al.* Antibody directed enzyme prodrug therapy (ADEPT): Clinical Report. *Disease Markers* 1991; **9**: 233

The design of prodrugs for antibody-directed enzyme prodrug therapy (ADEPT)

C. J. Springer[1]*, I. Niculescu-Duvaz[1],
A. B. Mauger[1], T. A. Connors[1], P. J. Burke[2],
D. H. Davies[3], R. I. Dowell[3], F. T. Boyle[3],
D. C. Blakey[3], R. G. Melton[4]

[1]CRC Centre for Cancer Therapeutics, Institute of Cancer Research, Cotswold Road, Surrey, [2]Medical Oncology Department, Charing Cross Hospital, London, [3]Cancer Research Department, Zeneca Pharmaceuticals, Macclesfield, [4]PHLS, CAMR, Porton Down, Wilts, UK

ADEPT (antibody directed enzyme prodrug therapy) is a hghly selective treatment for maximising tumour exposure to cytotoxic agents [1,2]. It involves the administration of a tumour-specific antibody that is conjugated to an enzyme. After a time interval to allow for localisation of the conjugate at the tumour and clearance of non-tumour bound conjugate from blood and other tissues, a prodrug is injected. The prodrug is then converted specifically to a cytotoxic drug by the enzyme localised at the tumour site. We have used the bacterial enzyme carboxypeptidase G2 (CPG2), to convert prodrugs (which are poor cytotoxic agents) to potent drugs. The drug is derivatised to the prodrug with a glutamic acid group which is cleaved by the enzyme in the conjugate.

Antibodies which bind to specific tumour antigens have been conjugated to CPG2. *In vivo* experiments with the benzoic acid mustard derived prodrugs, 4-[bis(2-chloroethyl)amino]benzoyl-L-glutamic acid (Figure 1) and

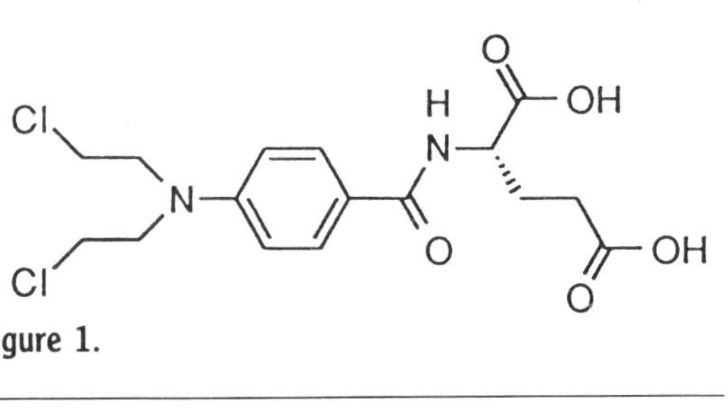

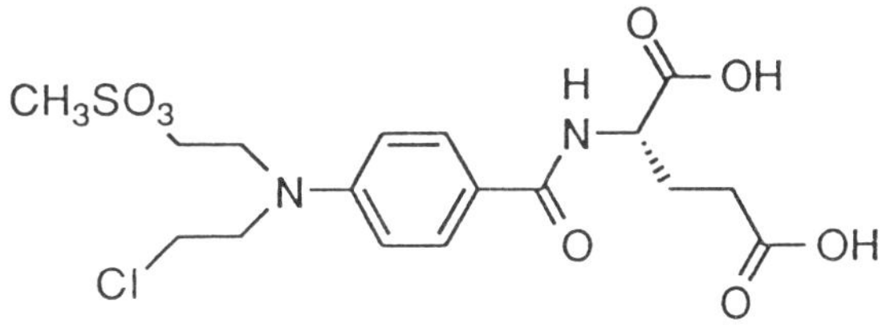

Figure 2.

4-[(chloroethyl)[2-(mesyloxy)ethyl]amino]benzoyl-L-glutamic acid (Figure 2), [3] have shown regressions in established choriocarcinoma and breast tumour xenografts [2,4,5].

These prodrugs are bifunctional alkylating agents in which the activating effect of the ionised carboxyl function is masked through an amide bond to the glutamic acid residue. The F(ab')₂ fragment of the mouse monoclonal antibody A5B7 has been conjugated to CPG2 and used with the prodrug 4-[(2-chloroethyl)[2-(mesyloxy)ethyl]amino] benzoyl-L-glutamic acid (Figure 2) in two clinical trials for colorectal carcinoma: a pilot scale ADEPT trial performed by Prof. K. Bagshawe at the Charing Cross Hospital [6] and an ongoing trial performed by Prof. R. Begent at the Royal Free Hospital.

A variety of different prodrugs have been made in order to determine the most effective prodrug for use in ADEPT. A large range of different aromatic nitrogen mustard prodrugs have been synthesised and analysed by *in vitro* criteria. Some of the favourable attributes sought in the prodrug/drug combination are:

Figure 1.

*Author to whom correspondence should be addressed.

1. Good enzyme kinetics in order to effect prodrug to drug conversion.
2. A short chemical half-life for the drug in order to avoid toxicity of normal tissues due to leak-back from the tumour site.
3. A potent activated drug.
4. A large toxicity separation between the prodrug and its corresponding activated drug.

The first series of prodrugs to be synthesised were the unsubstituted benzoic acid mustard glutamates (Figures 1–3). These vary in their different alkylating functionalities. All these prodrugs are good substrates for CPG2 and are cleaved to their correspondingly activated drugs (Figures 4–6) respectively [4].

The prodrugs are less reactive than their corresponding active drugs, as demonstrated by measuring the chemical half-life of each prodrug: $t_{1/2}$ 1158, 984 and 42 min for prodrugs (Figures 1, 2 and 3 respectively), compared to $t_{1/2}$ 324, 58, 21 min for the corresponding active drugs (Figures 4, 5 and 6 respectively) [7]. These prodrugs are

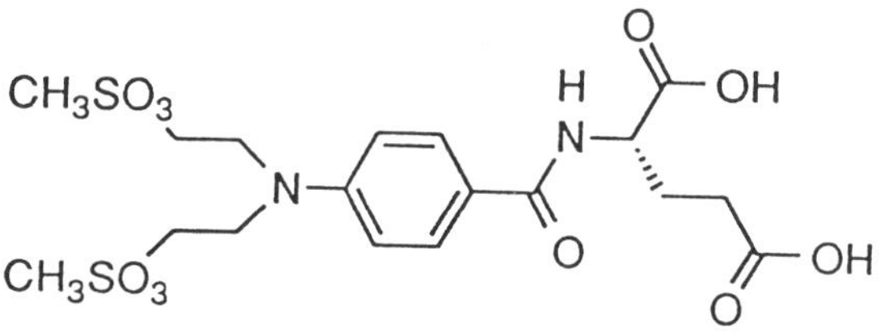

Figure 3.

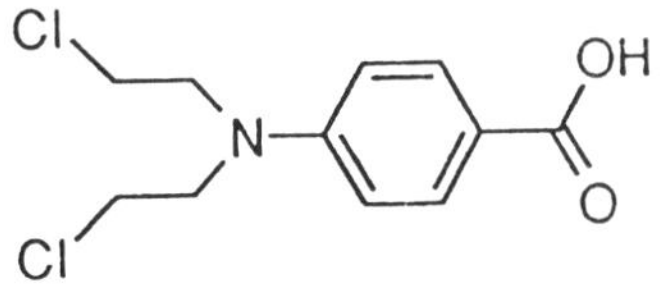

Figure 4.

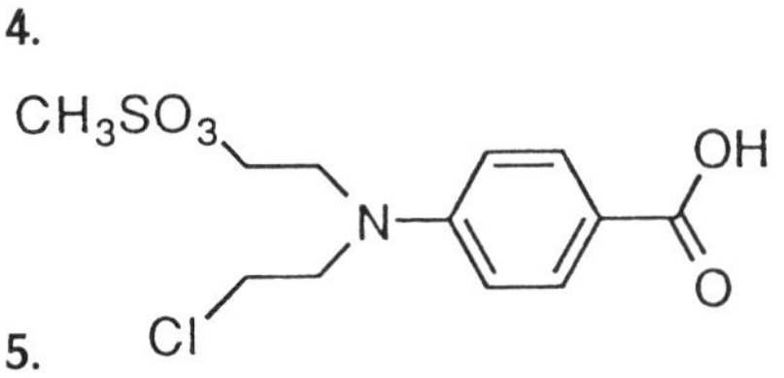

Figure 5.

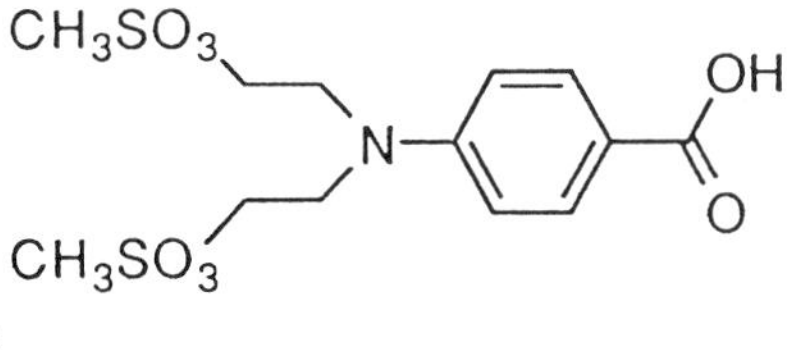

Figure 6.

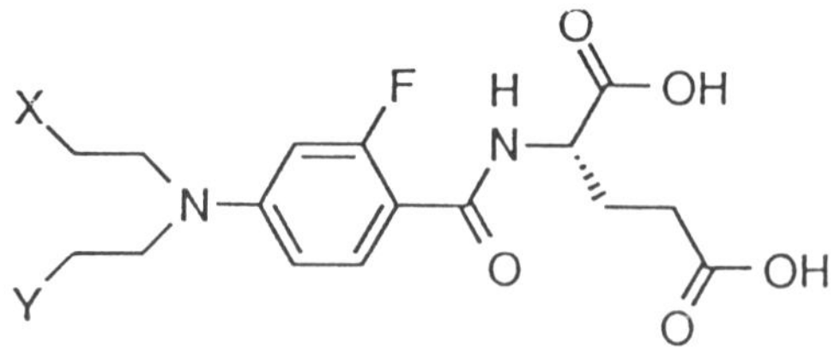

X, Y =Cl / CH₃SO₃

Figure 7.

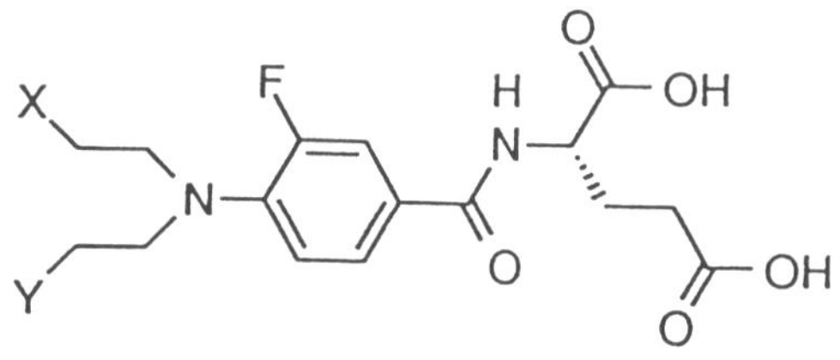

Figure 8.

non-toxic in cell cytotoxicity assays- $IC_{50} \gg 1000$ μM for 1 h incubation, and are activated to more toxic drugs of $IC_{50} \sim 200$ μM. Prodrug 2 which is activated to drug 5 is the system used in the therapy experiments and clinical trials referred to above.

All these prodrugs fulfil point 1 above (prodrugs with good kinetics for CPG2) stated as one of our goals. However, the half-life did not appear to be optimal with this class of compounds (point 2 above). Accordingly a range of compounds was designed with varying half-lives in order to develop prodrugs that are cleaved to active drugs that cannot leak-back from the tumour. Benzoic acid mustard prodrugs with fluorine-substituents in the 2- or 3- position on the benzene ring (Figures 7 and 8 respectively) were synthesised and the half-lives measured.

It was found that the 3-fluoro group had much shorter half-lives than their corresponding non-substituted compounds: $t_{1/2}$ 147 (cf. 1158), 122 (cf. 984) and 9 (cf. 42) min for the 3-fluoro benzoic acid prodrug groups (Figure 7), compared to $t_{1/2}$ 72 (cf. 324), 2.4 (cf. 58) and 1.9 (cf. 21) min for corresponding 3-fluoro drug groups. Although the criteria for short half-life drugs has been met, with this series the activated drugs fall short of our stated goals of potency (point 3 above), since the most potent drug still has an IC_{50} of > 200 μM [8].

To enhance efficacy in ADEPT, phenol mustard-prodrugs (Figure 9), and aniline-mustard-prodrugs (Figure 10), were synthesised which release much more potent phenol mustard- and aniline-mustard drugs [9–11].

Structural modifications were made to the mustard arms, to the aromatic ring and to the glutamate moiety

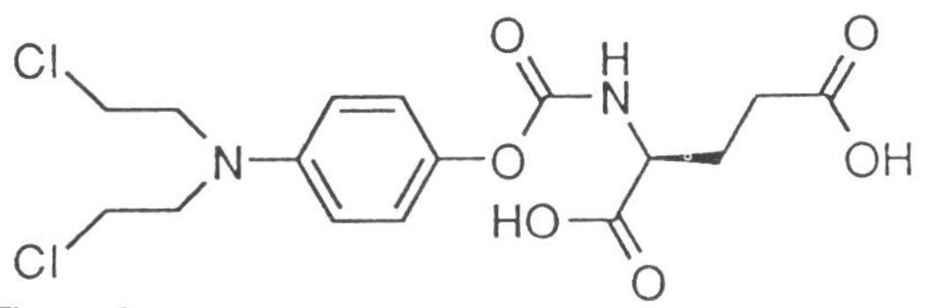

Figure 9.

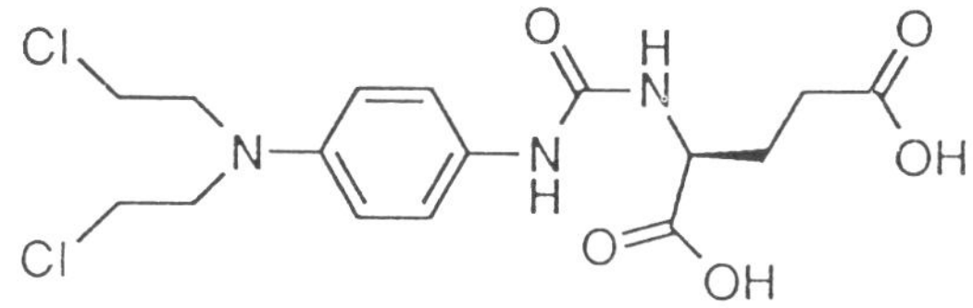

Figure 10.

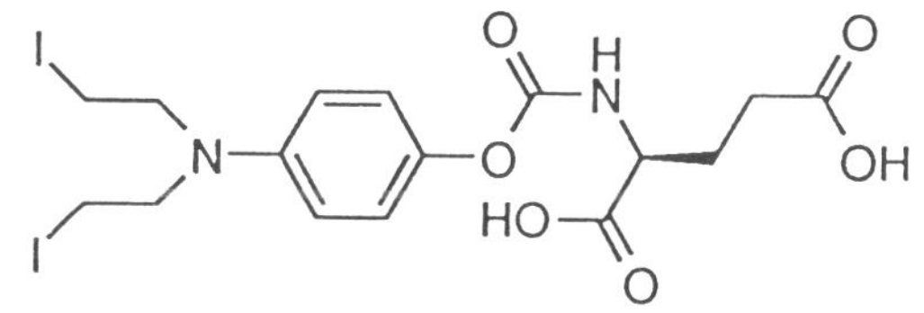

Figure 11.

[12,13]. Surprisingly, these prodrugs are substrates for the CPG2 enzyme (K_m 1–10 μM, k_{cat} 10–40 s⁻¹). The cytotoxicity of the active drugs (IC_{50} 0.5–10 μM) released by cleavage with CPG2 is considerably enhanced over that of the benzoic acid drugs. These novel drugs are > 50 fold more toxic than their corresponding prodrugs.

Recently, the efficacy of the prodrugs has been enhanced by the use of bisiodo-mustard arms in the phenol prodrug series (Figure 11) [14,15]. This prodrug (ZD2767P) is also a good substrate for the CPG2 enzyme (K_m 1 μM, k_{cat} 30 s⁻¹) and the active drug that is released with CPG2 is very potent in cytotoxicity assays (IC_{50} < 0.3 μM) which is over 100 fold more potent than the corresponding glutamate prodrug, 11. The half-life of the active drug is beneficially of the order of a few seconds thus minimising leak-back of active drug from the tumour.

These data indicate that prodrugs for ADEPT have been made for activation by CPG2 with different chemical and biochemical characteristics within the highly specific requirements of the CPG2 enzyme.

REFERENCES

1 Bagshawe KD. Antibody directed enzymes revive anti-cancer prodrugs concept. *Br J Cancer* 1987; **58**: 531–2

2 Bagshawe KD, Springer CJ, Searle F, *et al*. A Cytotoxic agent can be generated selectively at cancer sites. *Br J Cancer* 1988; **58**: 700–3

3 Springer CJ, Antoniw P, Bagshawe KD, Searle F, Bisset GMF, Jarman M. Novel prodrugs which are activated to cytotoxic alkylating agents by carboxypeptidase G2. *J Med Chem* 1990; **33**: 677–81

4 Springer CJ, Bagshawe KD, Sharma SK, *et al*. Ablation of human choriocarcinoma xenografts in nude mice by antibody-directed enzyme prodrug therapy (ADEPT) with three novel compounds. *Eur J Cancer* 1991; **27**: 1361–6

5 Eccles SA, Court WJ, Box GA, Dean CJ, Springer CJ. Regression of established breast carcinoma xenografts with antibody-directed enzyme prodrug therapy (ADEPT) against c-erbB₂ p185. *Cancer Res* 1994 (in press)

6 Bagshawe KD, Sharma SK, Springer CJ, *et al*. Antibody-enzyme conjugates can generate cytotoxic drugs from inactive precursors at tumor sites. *Antibody Immunoconjug Radiopharm* 1991; **4**: 915–22

7 Springer CJ, Antoniw P, Bagshawe KD, Wilman DEV. Comparison of half-lives and cytotoxicity of N-chloroethyl-4-amino and N-mesyloxyethyl-benzoyl compounds, products of prodrugs in antibody-directed enzyme prodrug therapy (ADEPT). *Anti-Cancer Drug Des* 1991; **6**: 467–79

8 Springer CJ, Niculescu-Duvaz I, Pedley RB. Novel prodrugs of alkylating agents derived from 2-fluoro- and 3-fluoro benzoic acids for antibody-directed enzyme prodrug therapy. *J Med Chem* 1994; **37**: 2361–70

9 Springer CJ, Burke PJ, Blakey DC, Davies DH, Dowell RI, Melton RG. Tumour regressions with novel prodrugs in antibody-directed enzyme prodrug therapy (ADEPT). *Eur J Cancer* 1994; **30A**: 59

10 Blakey DC, Davies DH, Dowell RI, *et al*. Anti-tumour effects of an aniline mustard used in antibody-directed enzyme prodrug therapy (ADEPT). *Br J Cancer* 1994; **69 (suppl XXI)**: 14

11 Blakey DC, Davies DH, Dowell RI, Burke PJ, Springer CJ, Melton RG. Anti-tumour effects of an antibody-carboxypeptidase g2 conjugate in combination with a phenol mustard prodrug. *Proc AACR* 1994; **35**: A3023, 507

12 Springer CJ, Burke PJ, Blakey DC, Davies DH, Dowell RI, Melton RM. Antitumour efficacy of novel prodrugs in antibody-directed enzyme prodrug therapy (ADEPT). *Antibody Immunoconjug Radiopharm* 1994; **7**: **49**

13 Davies DH, Dowell RI, Boyle FT, *et al*. New mustard prodrugs for ADEPT (antibody-directed enzyme prodrug therapy). *Annals Onc* 1994; **5 (suppl 5)**: 73

14 Springer CJ, Blakey DC, Mauger AG, *et al*. A novel bisiodo-phenol mustard prodrug for antibody-directed enzyme prodrug therapy (ADEPT). *Proc Advances in the Applications of Monoclonal Antibodies in Clinical Oncology*, Lesbos, Greece 1994; 41

15 Blakey DC, Springer CJ, Mauger AG, *et al*. Tumour regressions caused by a bis-iodo phenol mustard prodrug in antibody-directed enzyme prodrug therapy (ADEPT). *Proc Advances in the Applications of Monoclonal Antibodies in Clinical Oncology*, Lesbos, Greece 1994; 42

First pilot clinical trial of ADEPT

Kenneth D. Bagshawe

Emeritus Professor of Medical Oncology, Charing Cross and Westminster Medical School, London, UK

PHASE I STUDY OF PRODRUG CMDA

The study was carried out in two parts. In the first, prodrug was given alone to determine whether it posed any toxicity not revealed in rodents. There was evidence from mouse studies that intestinal contents showed carboxypeptidase G2 (CPG2)-like activity and if this were so in the human then there would be a case for incorporating gut sterilising antibiotics into the protocol. As the study proceeded it also became clear that a further benefit of studying the prodrug alone was determination of its plasma half-life in the absence of administered enzymes.

Seven patients entered the first part of the study. The prodrug designated CMDA (4-[(chlorethyl) (2 methyl oxy)ethyl] amino benzoyl-L-glutamic acid) was dissolved in dimethyl sulphoxide (DMSO) and immediately before administration it was diluted in 1.26% sodium bicarbonate and given as a slow i.v. bolus.

Five of the seven patients received one or more injections on one day, the other two received injections over three and six days. On the basis of experience with mouse xenografted with LS174T colorectal cancer six days post AEC seemed likely to be the maximum time that an effective concentration of enzyme would be available at tumour sites with CEA as the target antigen. The limited supply of prodrug restricted the range of prodrug that was given to a total of 0.2–2.4 G/m^2.

At these dose levels toxicity was absent or restricted to nausea and vomiting at the higher dose levels. In contrast to the mouse studies, high pressure liquid chromatography (HPLC) of plasma showed no evidence of active drug formation so that there was no indication for giving gut sterilising antibiotics in man. The mean half-life of the prodrug was 29.4 ± 4.8 min. and peak plasma concentrations were in the range of 15–50 µg/ml. There was no evidence of therapeutic effect and two of the seven patients were later judged too ill to proceed to the full ADEPT trial.

FIRST ADEPT TRIAL

The agents available were 1) the $F(ab')2$ fragment of antibody A5B7 directed at carcinoembryonic antigen (CEA) [1] conjugated to a bacterial enzyme, carboxypeptidase G2 (CPG2) [2]. 2) A second murine monoclonal antibody (SB43) which inactivates CPG2 and which was galactosylated to ensure rapid clearance from blood [3] and 3) the prodrug CMDA in a formulation which required administration in dimethyl sulphoxide (DMSO).

Animal studies had shown that if the CMDA prodrug was given in therapeutic dosage when the plasma enzyme level was > 0.3 enzyme units/ml fatal toxicity resulted from rapid activation of the prodrug. At 56–72 h post-AEC tumour enzyme levels were still high. Without accelerated clearance a safe level of plasma AEC was obtained in the mouse with LS174T xenografts only 6–7 days post AEC at which time tumour AEC had fallen to an ineffective concentration. In the mouse, bolus i.v. injections of SB43-gal had resulted in deaths presumptively attributed to immune complex formation.

OBJECTIVES

A first objective of the study was to determine the general feasibility of an approach in which agents interact with each other in the patient. There are many variables in the system and few guidelines for the translation of such a system from mouse to man. The variables include the dose of AEC and the its rate of administration; the time interval between AEC and the second antibody SB43-gal, the amount of SB43-gal, and, critically, the rate and duration of its administration; the times at which prodrug is given, its total dosage and fractionation, dose escalation and the issue of bolus versus constant infusion.

The rate of clearance of the AEC in the human was unknown and the safety of giving SB43-gal intravenously in the presence of circulating AEC was uncertain. On the basis of calculations based on mouse data the estimated requirement of SB43-gal was about 240 mg/m^2. It was also hoped to determine a level of plasma enzyme activity for safe administration of the prodrug. Since it seems unlikely that any cytotoxic agent will sterilise a cancer cell population of 10^{10}–10^{11} cells in a single 4–6 day cycle of therapy [4] it was also decided to see whether immunosuppression with cyclosporin would permit more than one cycle of therapy to be given.

MATERIALS, METHODS AND PATIENTS

Full details of materials and methods and patients with adenocarcinoma of the lower bowel will be published elsewhere [5]. In brief, the patients all had extensive, recurrent adenocarcinoma of lower bowel, after surgery and full conventional cytotoxic therapy with 5 fluorouracil and folinic acid.

Study Design

The patients were studied in three groups. Group 1 consisted of six patients who received 20000 enzyme units/m^2 in the AEC which was given as a 2-h i.v. infusion. Starting 46 h later an i.v. infusion of SB43-gal was given over a period of 3–5 h. Prodrug administration started 72 h after the start of the AEC infusion. The dose of SB43 given to the first patient (Case No. 2) was 240 mg/m^2. The rapid fall in plasma enzyme activity during this infusion indicated that smaller amounts could be given to subsequent patients.

Three patients received a total dose of < 1.5 g/m^2 of CMDA by slow i.v. bolus. Toxicity in these patients was slight or absent and therapeutic benefit was also slight or absent. The other three patients received 2.7–3.9 g/m^2 of CMDA over five days; all had nausea and vomiting during treatment and grade 4 myelotoxicity subsequently with full recovery within 25 days. At the time prodrug was started serum enzyme was < 0.02 enzyme units. The $t_{1/2}$ of the prodrug in plasma was shorter than in patients in the first

stage of the study who had not received AEC. Two of these three patients had partial remissions and one had a mixed response. The latter patient was known from his original histochemisty of biopsied lymph nodes to have both CEA positive and CEA negative metastases.

There were no toxic effects attributed to the AEC or SB43-gal infusions. The AEC level in plasma proved comparable to that found optimal for CMDA prodrug in the mouse. The rate of clearance of AEC in patients prior to SB43-gal was similar to that of the mouse.

Group 2

The objective in this group was to administer the prodrug by continuous i.v. infusion over a period of five days with the amount of AEC unchanged and SB43-gal in a dose similar to the later patients in Group 1. Prodrug dosage was similar to the higher doses used in Group 1 and was given over five days.

Technical difficulties resulted from the action of DMSO on various types of syringe so that the amount of CMDA received by the first patient in the group was less than planned. A further technical difficulty affected three other patients in this group in that they had little or no myelotoxicity and no therapeutic response. This was attributed to a batch of AEC which although satisfactory on formal testing for antigen binding and catalytic activity was subsequently found to show poor localisation in mouse xenografts. The one patient in this group who received the planned dose of CMDA (4 g/m^2) over five days had a partial response with grade 4 myelosuppression, disease progression recurring six months later with survival for 24 months.

During this study it was found that SB43-gal could be given over a longer period without loss of efficacy as judged by the fall in plasma enzyme activity.

Giving CMDA by slow infusion reduced the incidence and intensity of nausea and vomiting compared with bolus injections but this group gave us no indication of the efficacy of continuous infusion compared with bolus injections.

Group 3

The main objective in this final group of patients was to determine whether cyclosporin administration would delay the development of the host antibody response to both murine and bacterial antigens. Unfortunately, the next two patients referred for ADEPT both had massive hepatic metastases with liver margins at the pelvic brim and gross disturbance of hepatic function. However a previous patient (Case No. 5) had similar hepatic impairment and had tolerated treatment satisfactorily but had not received cyclosporin. Oral cyclosporin (400 mg 12-hourly) was started 48 h before the AEC infusion and the intention was to continue it through to a second cycle of therapy maintaining cyclosporin levels between 150–350 µg/l by dose adjustment according to cyclosporin blood levels. Cyclosporin blood levels fluctuated considerably during prodrug administration and following completion of the first cycle of therapy renal function deteriorated. Cyclosporin was discontinued but both patients developed Grade 4 myelosuppression and died with evidence of both renal and hepatic failure.

The remaining patients in Group 3 received 80 mg/m^2 cyclosporin in 5% dextrose by continuous infusion every 12 h with dose modification according to blood levels. This proved more satisfactory in maintaining blood levels within the target limits than the oral route.

A further series of changes were undertaken in the course of treating this group of patients. The duration of SB34-gal administration was prolonged and for the last three patients it was continued at a low rate throughout the period of prodrug administration. This was done on the basis that it seemed possible that small amounts of enzyme diffused back into the plasma from extra cellular fluid after the plasma enzyme had been depleted by SB43 and could activate the slowly infused prodrug before it reached tumour sites. Additionally, in the last three patients the amounts of conjugate given in their first two cycles of therapy was reduced to 5000 enzyme units/m^2 and this also may have contributed to the absence of serious myelotoxicity. The presence of low levels of anti-mouse and anti-bacterial antibodies before the third cycle of therapy in two cases led to increases in the dose of AEC with their final cycles of treatment. One patient with mucoid ascites from an appendix carcinoma and an anterior abdominal wall mass showed a marked reduction in both ascites and mass. The final case was febrile and had intractable pelvic pain, a third cycle of therapy was not given because of his general weakness. Following therapy there was a brief period of myelosuppression and his morphine requirement was greatly reduced for several weeks but there was no objective response.

This study of Group 3 indicated the danger of cyclosporin combined with chemotherapy in patients with severe impairment of hepatic function. It also showed that cyclosporin delayed the development of the human anti-mouse antibody (HAMA) and antibacterial enzyme response from about 9–10 days to 20–22 days, thus allowing three successive weekly cycles of ADEPT to be given. The absence of myelosuppression in two patients who received 7.9 and 9 g/m^2 of the CMDA prodrug which is more than three times the amount that produced grade 4 myelosuppression in the early part of the study indicates the importance of ensuring that the plasma is free of enzyme when prodrug is given.

The issue of whether the prodrug should be given by continuous i.v. infusion or bolus administration has not been resolved. If there is any enzyme in the plasma then it is probably advantageous to give the prodrug by bolus since it will saturate plasma enzyme and reach the tumour sites but if complete elimination of enzyme from plasma is achieved then the advantage of maximising the turnover of prodrug at tumour sites lies with its infusion.

This first trial with ADEPT has shown that it is possible to construct prodrugs that are essentially non-toxic. The general approach of using agents which interact *in vivo* is feasible and with an appropriate selection of patients can be carried out safely. Control of plasma enzyme levels is probably essential to avoid myelotoxicity with any prodrug and this can be achieved by means of a second antibody directed at the AEC.

Various factors in the referral pattern for the present study resulted in most of the patients having very advanced disease at the time of the treament. Eight patients received > 2.4 g/m^2 of CMDA or more and were assessible; four of those had partial responses and one had a mixed response. This suggests that with prodrugs that generate more active drugs than CMDA it should be possible to achieve a valuable form of therapy.

It remains to be determined whether new developments with antibody-enzyme constructs and new prodrugs avoid the necessity of eliminating enzyme from plasma.

Acknowledgments

I would like to thank Drs S. K. Sharma, C. J. Springer, P. Antoniw and R. Melton for making the agents and performing the measurements reported in the study.

REFERENCES

1 Harwood PJ, Britton DW, Southall PJ, *et al.* Mapping epitope characteristics on carcinoembryonic antigen. *Br J Cancer* 1986; **54**: 75–82

2 Sherwood RF, Melton RG, Alwan SM, *et al*. Purification and properties of carboxypeptidase G2 from pseudomonas strain RS 16. *Eur J Biochem* 1985; **148**: 447–53

3 Sharma SK, Bagshawe KD, Burke PJ, *et al*. Inactivation and clearance of an anti-CEA carboxypeptidase G2 conjugate in blood after localisation in a xenograft model. *Br J Cancer* 1990; **61**: 659–62

4 Springer CJ, Antoniw P, Bagshawe KD, *et al*. Novel prodrugs which are activated to cytotoxic alkylating agents by carboxypeptidase G2. *J Med Chem* 1990; **33**: 677–81

5 Bagshawe KD, Springer CJ, Sharma SK. Antibody-directed prodrug therapy: Pilot Scale Clinical Trial. 1994 (Submitted for publication)

ZD2767: A potent and selective system for antibody-directed enzyme prodrug therapy (ADEPT)

DC Blakey[1], DH Davies[1], RI Dowsell[1], SJ East[1], CJ Springer[2], AB Mauger[2], PJ Burke[3], and RH Melton[4]

[1]*Cancer Research Department, Zeneca Pharmaceuticals, Alderley Park, Cheshire,* [2]*Institute of Cancer Research, Sutton, Surrey,* [3]*Charing Cross Hospital, London and* [4]*PHLS, CAMR, Porton, UK*

Antibody-directed enzyme prodrug therapy (ADEPT) is a two-step targeting strategy for the treatment of cancer. We have developed an ADEPT system, ZD2767, consisting of a conjugate of the F(ab')$_2$ fragment of the anti-CEA antibody, A57, and carboxypeptidase G2 and a prodrug of p-[N,N-bis(2-iodoethyl)amino]phenol mustard and L-glutamic acid. Surprisingly the prodrug is a good substrate for CPG2 (km $\sim$ 1 μmol and kcat $\sim$ 30 s^{-1}) and cleavage releases the potent bis-iodo phenol mustard drug (IC50=0.3 μmol against LoVo cells). The ZD2767 conjugate localises to human LoVo colorectal tumour xenografts growing s.c. in athymic nude mice. Approximately 1%/g of injected ZD2767 conjugate remains at the tumour after 72 h and blood and normal tissue levels of the conjugate are 10–50 fold larger than those in the tumour at this time point. The ZD2767 prodrug (3 × 70 mg/kg given as 3 i.p. injections over 2 h) was administered 72 h after the administration of the ZD2767 conjugate (2.5 mg/kg i.v.) to athymic mice bearing established (6–7 mm diameter) LoVo tumour xenografts. This treatment schedule with ZD2767 resulted in approximately 50% of the tumours undergoing complete regressions, tumour growth delays > 30 days and little toxicity as judged by body weight loss (6–7%). These studies confirm the potential of this ADEPT system, ZD2767, for the treatment of colorectal cancer.

Use of a branched lysyl derivative of α-melanocyte stimulating hormone for targeting to melanoma

DR Bard
Strangeways Research Laboratory, Worts' Causeway, Cambridge CB1 4RN, UK

A compound, *bis*MSH-DTPA, based on the tridecapeptide, α-melanocyte stimulating hormone (MSH), (DTPA= diethylenetriaminepentaacetic acid) complexed with indium-111, has been shown to be an effective imaging agent for malignant melanoma in the clinic. More recently we have shown that compounds based on the heptapeptide MSH analogue, [Nle^4, ASP^5, *D*-Phe^7, ys^{10}]-α-MSH$_{(4–10)}$ show improved tumour localisation with less unspecific liver uptake. A potential problem in using such a system to deliver imaging or cytotoxic preparations to melanoma cells is that only a single molecule of the targeted agent can be delivered to each receptor.

We have therefore synthesised derivatives of MSH$_{(4–10)}$ in which the *N'*-terminus is extended by the addition of a branched lysyl construct separated from the main peptide by a spacer sequence constructed from two 4-aminobutyric acid moieties. This group had little effect on the biological activity of the peptide and enabled up to eight molecules of tyrosine to be attached to each MSH$_{(4–10)}$ sequence. These were then iodinated.

Uptake of these compounds *in vivo* showed a significant enhancement of tumour uptake compared with a single substituted MSH$_{(4–10)}$. Unspecific liver uptake was highly dependent on the lipophilicity of the peptide and was higher if the *N'*-terminal tyrosines were acetylated. These experiments indicate that branched polylysyl structures, enabling multiple substitution of a ligand, can be used to enhance receptor dependent uptake with minimal loss of biological activity.

^{32}P-labelled antibodies for radioimmunotherapy: recent developments and a preliminary report of the first Phase I studies

HA Band, AM Creighton, KE Britton, J Long, C Bartram and M Granowska

Department of Nuclear Medicine, St Bartholomew's Hospital, London EC1, UK

A method for labelling mononuclear antibodies with carrier-free ^{32}P gives products which allow the radionuclide to be targeted to tumours with appropriate antigens (Foxwell *et al. Br J Cancer* 1988). A simplified procedure is used to couple a phosphate-receptor peptide directly to the antibody for enzymatic phosphorylation with ^{32}P-ATP. The product is then separated on a Sepharose column using a semi-automatic FPLC system under sterile conditions with appropriate shielding. Radiochemical yields in clinical preparations have been about 40–50%. New purification procedures currently being adapted for clinical application should soon allow the use of a very much cheaper source of ^{32}P so that the radionuclide cost of a 10mCi dose would be about £100.

Four polycythaemic patients received single doses of from 1.9–5.5mCi i.v. (at 1.00–1.65mCi/mg) of ^{32}P-labelled SM3 in a pilot Phase I study. The labelled conjugate cleared from the circulation at a very similar rate to the corresponding macrocyclic ^{111}In-labelled antibody. There was no significant effect on haemoglobin, white cells or blood chemistry but in two patients with high platelets receiving about 5mCi or ^{32}P-SM3, a significant reduction in platelets was observed to normal levels. In a second study involving hepatic metastases from colorectal primaries, the first two patients were treated with 2.4–5.0mCi of ^{32}P-labelled PR1A3 intra-arterially (at 0.74–1.00mCi/mg) without untoward effect. Good stability was again achieved and in one case a second treatment of 5mCi was given four months later. A fall in serum CEA was noted but with an increase in tumour size.

^{32}P has optimal properties for radioimmunotherapy (Britton *et al. Nucl Med Commun* 1991; Rao & Howell, *J Nucl Med* 1993). The way appears to be clear for the evaluation of ^{32}P-labelled antibodies in the treatment of cancers.

Enhanced tumour specificity of an anti-carcinoembryonic antigen Fab' fragment by polyethylene glycol (PEG) modification

Cristina Delgado[1], R Barbara Pedley[2], Robert Boden[2], Joan A Boden[2], Patricia A Keep[2], Kerry A Chester[2], Derek Fisher[1], Richard HJ Begent[2] and Gillian E Francis[1]

[1]*Molecular Cell Pathology,* [2]*Targeting and Imaging Group, Royal Free Hospital School of Medicine, Rowland Hill Street, London NW3, UK*

Polyethylene glycol (PEG) modification of proteins alters their pharmacokinetics and biodistribution and has been reported to enhance tumour localisation of antibodies raised against tumour antigens, but the mechanism for the latter is obscure. Here we demonstrate that PEG-modification of a Fab' fragment (F9) of A5B7 (α-CEA) using an improved coupling method, increases its specificity for subcutaneous LS174T tumours implanted in TO nude mice. Although the area under the curve values (AUC) for PEG-F9 exceeded those for F9 in all tissues, there was a larger proportional increment in the AUC for the tumour than for normal tissues and hence an improvement in therapeutic index is anticipated. This was achieved despite a moderate loss in antigen binding of PEG-F9. In order to exploit these findings in tumour targeting, insight is required into the way in which PEG-modification influences biodistribution. We have examined the direction and rate of change in various informative ratios (such as tumour to tissue ratios and PEG-F9:F9 ratios) to gain insights into the influence of PEG on the transfer of the antibody into and out of normal tissues and the tumour. This reveals that the improved tumour uptake of antibody, achieved by PEG-modification, results from complex effects, influencing both the tumour and normal tissues and both entry into and exit from these sites.

Note: This work has been supported by Cancer Research Campaign.

Therapy of human B-cell lymphoma-bearing SCID mice is more effective with anti-CD19 and anti-CD38-saporin immunotoxins used in combination than with either immunotoxin used alone

David J Flavell, D Boehm and SU Flavell
The Simon Flavell Leukaemia Research Laboratory, University Department of Pathology, Southampton General Hospital, Southampton SO9 4XY, UK

An approach to overcoming the problem of heterogeneity of target antigen expression within a tumour cell population would be to target against two or more different surface antigens in the expectation that tumour cells that were multiple antigen negative would occur with a lower frequency than single antigen negative tumour cells. This strategy would not only improve the likelihood of delivering the cytotoxic agent to all cells within the tumour, but would also ensure delivery of greater amounts of the agent to those tumour cells that express all the target antigens.

We have explored the therapeutic effectiveness of administering anti-CD19-saporin (BU12-Sap) and anti-CD38-saporin (OKT10-Sap) immunotoxins (IT) either individually or in combination to SCID mice bearing the human Burkitt's lymphoma cell line RAMOS. Individual therapy groups consisted of 10 animals each (5 males, 5 females). Each group received 2×10^6 RAMOS cells i.v. injections administered on consecutive days commencing seven days after injection of tumour cells. All control animals receiving three sham injections of 200 µl PBS had

died with disseminated disease by 40 days with a median survival of 36 days. Animals receiving 10 µg BU12Sap IT × 3 had a median survival of 60 days and all animals in this group were dead by 69 days. BU12-Sap and OKT10=Sap ITs given in combination (5 µg of each IT × 3) led to a highly significant prolongation of survival with 30% of animals still alive and well at 150 days.

These studies show a significant improvement to *in vivo* therapeutic efficacy when saporin is delivered simultaneously against both CD19 and CD38 to RAMOS tumour cells compared with the very limited therapeutic effect that is seen when saporin is delivered against just one of these target molecules. It is speculated that the enhanced therapeutic effect obtained from using a combination of two different ITs results firstly from the delivery of greater amounts of saporin to double antigen positive RAMOS cells and secondly to the elimination of tumour cells that are single antigen negative that would otherwise escape destruction and result in tumour outgrowth when a single immunotoxin is used.

Isolation of tumour cell-associated single-chain Fvs from immunised mice using phage-antibody libraries and the reconstruction of whole antibodies from these antibody fragments

Catherine A Kettleborough[1], Keith H Ansell[1], Richard W Allen[1], Elisabet Rossell-Vives[2], Detlef H Güssow[2] and Mary M Bendig[1]

[1]MRC Collaborative Centre, 1–3 Burtonhole Lane, Mill Hill, London NW7 1AD, UK and [2]Laboratorio de Bioinvesticación, Merck-Igoda SA Caspe 108, 08080 Barcelona, Spain

Enhanced expression of epidermal growth factor receptor (EGFR) occurs on a variety of malignant tissues thus making anti-EGFR antibodies possible agents for the diagnosis and therapy of human tumours. Standard hybridoma technology has been used successfully to isolate anti-EGFR antibodies from immunised mice and rats. This presentation demonstrates that phage-antibody libraries are an alternative, and more versatile, method for isolating antibodies from immunised mice. Anti-EGFR antibodies were isolated from phage-antibody libraries constructed not only from the spleen of an immunised mouse but also from the draining lymph node of an immunised mouse and from *in vitro* immunised cells. Two of the single-chain Fvs (scFvs) isolated from the phage-antibody libraries were engineered to create partially humanised whole antibody molecules.

Human recombinant single chain or Fab fragments against members of the human CEA family: antigen specificity and distribution in epithelial tumour cell lines

P Jantscheff[1], J Embleton[2], G Nagel[1], G Winter[3] and F Grunert[1]

[1]Institute of Immunobiology, University of Freiburg, Germany; [2] Paterson Institute for Cancer Research, University of Manchester and [3]Cambridge Centre for Protein Engineering, Medical Research Council Centre, Cambridge, UK

Using a naive human cDNA library derived from the mRNA of blood lymphocytes of non-immunised donors we obtained recombinant human single chain fragments (scFvs) and Fab fragments and cloned them into phagemid vectors. Rescued phage particles were originally selected by panning on a crude CD66/CEA preparation.

Specificity of the 'antibody fragments' was determined by FACScan analysis using HeLa- or CHO-transfectants expressing various members of CD66/CEA family. The scFv's, a parental and two light chain shuffled offsprings, bound specifically only to CD66a/BGP, whereas the Fab bound to at least four of the transfectants.

The recognised epitope(s) could be localised in the N-domain of the CD66-molecules. Low or no binding was found to resting granulocytes (PMN), although the cells express CD66a, CD66c, and CD66d on their surface. But binding could be demonstrated after activation of granulocytes with the chemotactic active peptide n-formyl-Met-Leu-Phe (fMLP).

In FACScan analysis we could show that this epitope(s) is also expressed on surface of tumour cells from different cell lines. Surprisingly, in several tumour cell lines, the scFv-recognised 'BGP epitope' was present on a GPI-anchored molecule that was sensitive to PI-PLC treatment.

Production of a combinatorial antibody library to membrane-bound gangliosides in melanoma cells

Helen Jones[1,2], Eryl Liddell[2], Richard Allmann[1] and Reg Fish[1]

[1]*Research Laboratories, Velindre NHS Trust Hospital, Cardiff CF4 7XL and *[2]*Monoclonal Antibody Unit, School of Molecular and Medical Biosciences, University of Wales College Cardiff, PO Box 911, Cardiff CF1 3US, UK*

In patients with advanced melanoma, polysialylated gangliosides (e.g. GD3) are overexpressed. This overexpression and shedding of acidic glycosphingolipids into the extracellular spaces and blood may be factors involved in increased tumour growth, lack of immune cell recognition, angiogenesis and metastatic tumour spread. As a prerequisite to investigations concerned with some of these phenomena, we have attempted to produce monoclonal antibodies to a number of gangliosides. A combinatorial antibody library has been made from mice immunised with the human melanoma cell line SK-Mel 28, that is known to overexpress GD3. Using phage display techniques a range of different antibody fragments has been isolated from this library. These have been screened using ELISA, FACS analysis, and immunohistochemistry and are currently being characterised with respect to their binding to the commercially available gangliosides, GD3, GM3, GM2, GD2, GD1a, GD1b and GT1b, purified from bovine brain and to the gangliosides expressed on the melanoma cell lines SK-Mel 28, SK-Mel 19, SK-Mel 64, V39, and A375. The results of this characterisation will be presented.

Diagnostic and therapeutic potential and radiolabelled methylene blue for disseminated melanoma

Eva M Link

Department of Molecular Pathology, University College London Medical School, London W1P 6DB, UK

Almost random metastatic dissemination of melanoma causes main difficulties in the neoplasm's management. Systemic treatment selectively directed at melanoma, such as targeted radiotherapy, seems to be the most promising option among those presently available. Since melanoma is a pigmented tumour, melanin constitutes a suitable target for a radioisotope's carrier to be addressed to cells of the tumour. Methylene blue (MTB) possesses exceptionally high affinity to melanin and, therefore, if labelled with appropriate radioisotopes, reveals both a diagnostic and therapeutic potential for melanoma. ^{211}At-MTB (α-particle emitter) is very effective therapeutically as determined by the growth rate of cutaneous lesions and the size and number of metastases in lymph nodes and lungs. Its i.v. injection prevents a metastatic spread by scavenging melanoma cells circulating with blood (including those with low melanin content). No treatment-related pathology in normal organs has been found.

Gamma-camera and SPECT biodistribution studies of iodinated MTB in melanoma patients, and measurements of radioactivity content in biopsies, confirmed a high and stable uptake of MTB in melanoma metastases (tumour/surrounding tissue ratio=9 at 19–26 h after a single i.v. injection). Whole-body scans with gamma-camera enabled a detection of small (<1 cm) unsuspected metastases verified later by other methods. The results justify the introduction of radiolabelled MTB for early diagnosis and treatment of small melanoma metastases, as well as a prevention of metastatic spread of the tumour in man.

Phase I clinical studies with a monoclonal antibody directed against the human EGF receptor

H Modjtahedi[1], M Nicolson[2], T Hickish[2], S Eccles[1], L Jackson[1], J Moore[2], L Spencer[2], J Salter[2], J Sloane[2], M Gore[2], CJ Dean[1] and I Smith[1,2]
[1]Section of Immunology, Institute of Cancer Research and [2]Royal Marsden Hospital, Sutton and London, UK

Overexpression of the EGF receptor accompanied by production of its ligands (EGF, TGFα, amphiregulin) has been reported in a wide range of human malignancies including cancers of the breast, bladder, lung, brain, oesophagus and pancreas. High levels of expression of this receptor were associated with poor survival in many of these patients. We have produced a series of rat monoclonal antibodies (mAbs) to the external domain of EGF receptor using as immunogen the breast tumour cell line MDA-MB 468 which overexpresses the EGF receptor. Of these, mAb ICR62(IgG2b) was outstanding. This antibody, which binds to epitope C on the external domain of EGF receptor, is very effective in (1) blocking the binding of ligands (EGF, TGFα) to the EGFR on breast, brain, bladder, lung and head and neck carcinoma cells, and (2) inhibiting the growth of these tumours in vitro. More importantly, mAb ICR62 is very effective in eradicating EGFR overexpressing tumours grown as xenografts in athymic mice (Modjtahedi et al. Br J Cancer 1993; **67**: 254–61).

A phase I toxicity trial with this antibody was undertaken in the Royal Marsden Hospital in 20 patients (13 male and 7 female) with squamous carcinoma of the head and neck or lung which expressed the EGF receptor. Doses of up to 100 mg have been administered i.v. without untoward toxicity. Only 3/15 patients showed HARA responses. In patients receiving doses greater than 40 mg of ICR62, biopsies of metastatic lesions taken 24 h following treatment have shown good localisation of mAb ICR62. We conclude that mAb ICR62 which acts as a TGFα and EGF antagonist and localises efficiently to metastatic sites in patients with squamous cell carcinoma, may be useful for therapeutic applications in the significant number of cancer patients whose tumours overexpress the EGF receptor.

Identification of the epitope on carcinoembryonic antigen (CEA) defined by the antibody PR1A3

LMD Stewart[1], S Young[1], H Durbin[2], P Bates[3], D Snary[1] and WF Bodmer[2]
[1]Applied Development Laboratory, [2]Cancer Genetics and [3]Biomolecular Modelling, Imperial Cancer Research Fund, UK

The monoclonal antibody PR1A3 is used successfully for in vivo imaging of colorectal cancers, and the antigen has been identified as CEA. The antibody is particularly good in imaging since it does not bind circulating CEA and appears to be tumour specific. In order to determine the location of the PR1A3 epitope within CEA, a series of hybrid proteins were constructed using CEA and a structurally related protein, biliary glycoprotein (VGP). These studies demonstrated the last domain of CEA (B3) and the glycosyl-phosphatidylinositol (GPI) anchor are involved in antibody binding. Further studies involving expression of soluble constructs containing various domains fused to the Fc portion of an antibody, indicate that the GPI anchor may not be necessary for PR1A3 binding but may serve to distance the B3 domain from the membrane and allow antibody access.

Models of the combining site of the antibody indicate that there may be important charge interactions between the antibody and antigen. Using information obtained from these models and sequence comparisons with other family members, we have made CEA constructs containing mutations in key residues in the B3 domain of CEA and examined PR1A3 binding. The results of these studies may explain unique clinical properties exhibited by this antibody.

Construction, expression and purification of a carboxypeptidase G$_2$ anti-CEA scFv fusion protein for use in ADEPT

Paul Michael[1], Kerry Chester[2], Richard Begent[2], Roger Melton[1], Roger Sherwood[1] and Nigel Minton[1]

[1]*Department of Molecular Microbiology, Research Division, Centre for Applied Microbiology and Research, Porton Down, Salisbury, Wilts SP4 0JG, and* [2]*CRC Clinical Research Laboratories, Royal Free Hospital School of Medicine, Department of Clinical Oncology, Rowland Street, London NW3 2PF, UK*

There is, currently, considerable interest in the specific targeting of therapeutic agents to cancer cells. One particularly promising approach is a technique known as 'Antibody-directed enzyme prodrug therapy' (ADEPT). In this approach to cancer treatment an enzyme is coupled to a tumour-specific antibody, targeted to a tumour site and acts to release a highly cytotoxic drug from a subsequently administered, non-toxic prodrug. The use of the pseudomonad enzyme carboxypeptidase G$_2$ (CPG$_2$) with antibodies directed against carcinoembryonic antigen (CEA), has been at the forefront of ADEPT. Genetic fusion of the N-terminus of CPG$_2$ to the C-terminus of the light chain variable domain in a recombinant plasmid encoding a high affinity anti-CEA scFv, has been performed. An active fusion protein has been expressed and purified from *Escherichia coli*, with both enzyme and CEA binding activity. Characterisation of this fusion protein is at an early stage and assessment of its purification, yield, stability and pharmacokinetics is required if genetic fusion is to be considered as an alternative to chemical conjugation.

Ex-vivo identification of colorectal cancer lymph node metastases using the [124]I labelled anti-CEA monoclonal antibody A5B7: comparison with conventional histology and immunohistochemical techniques

GL Smith, RW Stirling, NA Theodorou and PM Dawson
Departments of Surgery and Histopathology, West Middlesex University Hospital, Twickenham Road, Isleworth, Middlesex TW7 6AF, UK

Colorectal cancer can be accurately localised peroperatively using a hand-held cadmium telluride probe (Neoprobe 100 TM) which detects radiolabelled monoclonal antibodies against carcinoembryonic antigen. We have evaluated the applicability of this technique to detection of lymph node metastases *ex-vivo*.

Thirty lymph nodes from 11 patients undergoing surgery for colorectal cancers were examined. Patients received intravenous ^{125}I-labelled anti-CEA monoclonal antibody (A5B7) prior to surgery. Following resection, the probe was used to detect labelled antibody within lymph nodes retrieved from the specimen. Nodes were stained by immunohistochemistry using anti-CEA antibodies and the second generation anti-TAG 72 antibody CC49. The probe counts and the immunohistochemical techniques were then compared with conventional histology to determine their accuracy in detection of nodal metastases.

The probe count accurately predicted histology in 83% of the nodes evaluated. There was no significant difference in accuracy between the probe technique and CEA immunohistochemistry (accuracy 80%). Both of these techniques were, however, more accurate than CC49 immunohistochemistry (accuracy 57%). This difference was statistically significant for the probe technique ($P < 0.05$ chi squared test).

The use of a hand held gamma detector in the *ex-vivo* assessment of lymph node metastases is feasible and is as accurate as conventional anti-CEA immunohistochemistry and more accurate than CC49 immunohistochemistry. This suggests that A5B7 is more suitable than CC49 for detection of colorectal cancer. This approach to lymph node staging merits further evaluation.

Comparison of distribution of F(AB')² A5B7 antibodies to CEA with and without flavone acetic acid in radio-immunotherapy of colorectal cancer

MP Napier, DM Lane, L Hope-Stone, AJ Green, JL Casey, PA Keep and RHJ Begent
CRC Laboratories, Department of Clinical Oncology, Royal Free Hospital School of Medicine, London, UK

By using a fragment of the mouse monoclonal antibody (F(ab')²), more efficient early uptake in tumour was seen compared to intact IgG. However, gamma camera studies of the distribution of ^{131}I-labelled antibody in tumour and normal tissue showed that whilst the peak uptake of antibody was at 4 h after administration, the clearance from the tumour was relatively rapid after that. If it were possible to maintain radiolabelled antibodies longer in the tumour, treatment would be more effective. Agents damaging tumour vasculature and reducing blood flow such as flavone acetic acid (FAA)—a synthetic compound based on the flavonoid aglycone ring structure—might improve this by trapping previously administered radiolabelled antibody in tumours. The purpose of this study was to test this hypothesis in patients.

Nine patients (11 therapies) received F(ab')² fragment of A5B7 antibody to CEA conjugated with 2035 Mbq/m² of ^{131}I and were compared to five patients (seven therapies) who received the same antibody followed 6 h later by an intravenous infusion of FAA (4.8 g/m² in 500 ml of 0.9% saline). The distribution was measured by quantitative SPECT gamma camera imaging.

The mean clearance from tumour in those patients who received F(ab')² A5B7 alone was 65.8 ± 19.9 h and 63.09 ± 18.5 h in those who received FAA as well (difference not significant). There was no significant difference in the cumulative radiation dose per unit of administered activity for tumour between the two groups.

Haematological toxicity was more severe in the FAA group with thrombocytopenia Grade I: 11% (F(ab')²) vs 43% (F(ab')²+FAA), Grade II: 0% vs 14%, Grade III: 11% vs 14% and Grade IV: 0% vs 29%, leucopenia Grade I: 22% vs 43% and Grade II: 0% vs 14%.

FAA did not enhance tumour retention of radiolabelled antibody in our study.